T0324174

Springer Theses

Recognizing Outstanding Ph.D. Research

Aims and Scope

The series "Springer Theses" brings together a selection of the very best Ph.D. theses from around the world and across the physical sciences. Nominated and endorsed by two recognized specialists, each published volume has been selected for its scientific excellence and the high impact of its contents for the pertinent field of research. For greater accessibility to non-specialists, the published versions include an extended introduction, as well as a foreword by the student's supervisor explaining the special relevance of the work for the field. As a whole, the series will provide a valuable resource both for newcomers to the research fields described, and for other scientists seeking detailed background information on special questions. Finally, it provides an accredited documentation of the valuable contributions made by today's younger generation of scientists.

Theses are accepted into the series by invited nomination only and must fulfill all of the following criteria

- They must be written in good English.
- The topic should fall within the confines of Chemistry, Physics, Earth Sciences, Engineering and related interdisciplinary fields such as Materials, Nanoscience, Chemical Engineering, Complex Systems and Biophysics.
- The work reported in the thesis must represent a significant scientific advance.
- If the thesis includes previously published material, permission to reproduce this must be gained from the respective copyright holder.
- They must have been examined and passed during the 12 months prior to nomination.
- Each thesis should include a foreword by the supervisor outlining the significance of its content.
- The theses should have a clearly defined structure including an introduction accessible to scientists not expert in that particular field.

More information about this series at http://www.springer.com/series/8790

Yu Chen

Design, Synthesis, Multifunctionalization and Biomedical Applications of Multifunctional Mesoporous Silica-Based Drug Delivery Nanosystems

Doctoral Thesis accepted by
Chinese Academy of Sciences, P.R. China

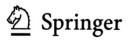 Springer

Author
Dr. Yu Chen
Shanghai Institute of Ceramics
Chinese Academy of Sciences
Shanghai
P.R. China

Supervisor
Prof. Jianlin Shi
Shanghai Institute of Ceramics
Chinese Academy of Sciences
Shanghai
P.R. China

ISSN 2190-5053   ISSN 2190-5061   (electronic)
Springer Theses
ISBN 978-3-662-48620-7   ISBN 978-3-662-48622-1   (eBook)
DOI 10.1007/978-3-662-48622-1

Library of Congress Control Number: 2015951802

Springer Heidelberg New York Dordrecht London

Printed on acid-free paper

Springer-Verlag GmbH Berlin Heidelberg is part of Springer Science+Business Media
(www.springer.com)

Parts of this thesis have been published in the following journal articles:

(1) Yu Chen, Hangrong Chen, Limin Guo, Qianjun He, Feng Chen, Jian Zhou, Jingwei Feng and Jianlin Shi, Hollow/Rattle-type Mesoporous Nanostructures by a Structural Difference-Based Selective Etching Strategy, *ACS Nano*, 2010, 4, 529–539.

(2) Yu Chen, Hangrong Chen, Deping Zeng, Yunbo Tian, Feng Chen, Jingwei Feng and Jianlin Shi, Core/Shell Structured Hollow Mesoporous Nanocapsules: A Potential Platform for Simultaneous Cell Imaging and Anticancer Drug Delivery, *ACS Nano*, 2010, 4, 6001–6013.

(3) Yu Chen, Hangrong Chen, Yang Sun, Yuanyi Zheng, Deping Zeng, Faqi Li, Shengjian Zhang, Xia Wang, Kun Zhang, Ming Ma, Qianjun He, Linlin Zhang and Jianlin Shi, Multifunctional Mesoporous Composite Nanocapsules for Highly Efficient MRI-Guided High Intensity Focused Ultrasound Cancer Surgery, *Angew. Chem. Int. Ed.*, 2011, 50, 12505–12509.

(4) Yu Chen, Hangrong Chen, Shengjian Zhang, Feng Chen, Lingxia Zhang, Jiamin Zhang, Min Zhu, Huixia Wu, Jingwei Feng and Jianlin Shi, Multifunctional Mesoporous Nanoellipsoids for Biological Bimodal Imaging and Magnetically Targeted Delivery of Anticancer Drugs, *Adv. Funct. Mater.*, 2011, 2, 270–278.

(5) Yu Chen, Chen Chu, Yuchuan Zhou, Hangrong Chen, Feng Chen, Qianjun He, Yonglian Zhang, Linlin Zhang and Jianlin Shi, Reversible Pore-Structure Evolution in Hollow Silica Nanocapsules: Large Pores for siRNA Delivery and Nanoparticle Collecting, *Small*, 2011, 7, 2935–2944.

(6) Yu Chen, Yu Gao, Hangrong Chen, Deping Zeng, Yaping Li, Yuanyi Zheng, Faqi Li, Xia Wang, Feng Chen, Qianjun He, Linlin Zhang and Jianlin Shi, Engineering "Inorganic Nanoemulsion/Nanoliposome" by Fluoride-Silica Chemistry for Efficient Delivery/Co-delivery of Hydrophobic Agents, *Adv. Funct. Mater.*, 2012, 22, 1586–1597.

Supervisor's Foreword

It is my great pleasure to introduce and recommend Dr. Yu Chen's research work for publication in the series of Springer Theses. His research work focuses on the design, synthesis, and biomedical applications of mesoporous silica-based nanosystems, under my supervision.

My research group devoted great efforts in developing new drug delivery systems (DDSs) for enhancing the chemotherapeutic efficiency of anticancer drugs. Mesoporous silica nanoparticles (MSNs) are one of the most promising nanocarriers among various organic and inorganic biomaterials due to their large surface area, high pore volume, tunable pore size, abundant surface chemistry, and high biocompatibility. We have been engaged in this research area for more than 10 years. In 2003, we successfully developed a soft-templating strategy to fabricate hollow mesoporous silica nanoparticles (HMSNs), which exhibited high drug-loading capacity. However, these HMSNs were severely aggregated with very poor dispersity. Therefore, the in vivo application and further clinical translation of these HMSNs were significantly restricted because of lacking suitable methods to obtain HMSNs with high dispersity and controllable parameters.

After joining my group, Dr. Chen's research focused on the development of a new synthetic methodology to fabricate HMSNs with desirable structure, morphology, and composition that are suitable for drug delivery in biomedicine. At the beginning of his research, he innovatively developed a new "structure difference-based selective etching" strategy to synthesize HMSNs with high dispersity and high drug-loading capacity. This new method employs the differences in condensation degree and structural-stability between solid silica nanoparticles and MSNs to selectively etch the inner core and thus produce the hollow interior afterwards. This method is very facile and environment-friendly, by which HMSNs can be synthesized on a large scale. The particle size of HMSNs can be tuned by changing the corresponding particle size of initial solid silica core, and the mesopore size of the shell can be controlled from 2.0 to more than 10 nm by selecting adequate etching duration. Importantly, this synthetic strategy can be extended to fabricate rattle-type multifunctional hollow mesoporous nanoparticles for thera-nostic applications against cancer, such as concurrent magnetic resonance imaging and anticancer drug delivery.

Furthermore, Dr. Chen systematically explored the biomedical applications of HMSNs, especially in ultrasound therapy. He developed HMSNs as the carriers to deliver hydrophobic perfluocarbon molecules for synergistic cancer surgery of high intensity focused ultrasound (HIFU). This is the first report on the development of new organic–inorganic hybrid nanosystems as the synergistic agents for enhanced HIFU ablation of tumors. Dr. Chen also functionalized HMSNs with manganese oxide nanoparticles for magnetic resonance imaging-guided HIFU cancer surgery. The biocompatibility and biological effects of as-synthesized HMSNs were also systematically investigated to promote the clinical applications of HMSNs.

Part of Dr. Chen's research has been published in high-impact journals such as Angew. Chem. Int. Ed., ACS Nano, Small, etc. The publication of this thesis in Springer is believed to promote scientific research in the community of materials science and medicine, especially in combating cancers based on nanobiotechnology and nanomedicine.

Shanghai   Prof. Jianlin Shi
June 2015

Acknowledgments

Recalling the past 5 years of pursuing my Ph.D. degree, I have abundant emotions bearing in mind. I have so many expectations in mind after the transformation from a Ph.D. student to a non-mature young scientific researcher. During the past 20 years of study, I have got plenty of help, encouragement, supervision, and guidance from my teachers, friends, and relatives. I greatly appreciate them, and I want to work harder to make great achievements in response to their help and expectations.

I want to express my thanks to my motherland. She has provided me the learning and growth opportunity and platform. Although there exists a large development gap between China and the developed countries, I strongly believe that the Chinese people will make our motherland stronger and more prosperous by virtue of the Chinese long-history tradition of hard work and wisdom. I also want to contribute as much as I can to realize this great goal.

I also want to express my sincere appreciation to my supervisor, Prof. Jianlin Shi, an outstanding scientist in materials science and chemistry. Professor Shi set an outstanding example in my life with his profound knowledge, rigorous and realistic attitude for research, noble character, and innovative-academic thinking. On the occasion of the completion of this thesis, I want to express the highest respect and heartfelt thanks to my supervisor for his hard training, teaching, cultivation, and help. I will remember his supervision, and will live up to his expectations. Meanwhile, I want to sincerely thank Prof. Hangrong Chen, my second supervisor. Professor Chen not only provided the guidance for my academic research, but also helped me a lot in my daily life. I want to convey my highest respect and heartfelt thanks to my beloved Prof. Chen.

The group members from Mesoporous and Low-dimensional Material Group in Shanghai Institute of Ceramics, Chinese Academy of Sciences also helped me a lot in the work and life. These members are Wenbo Bu, ZileHua, Lingxia Zhang, Lei Li, Weiming Huang, Xiangzhi Cui, Qianjun He, and Chengyang Wei. Thank you for the great support. In addition, I want to thank the students in the group, including Huixia Wu, Zhu Shu, Liming Guo, Fangming Cui, Jinjin Zhao,

Shaozong Zeng, Jian Zhou, Ze Gao, Zhengqing Ye, Nan Wang, Feng Chen, Jiaqi Li, Min Zhu, Huaiyong Xing, Jianan Liu, Lijun Wang, Yan Zhu, Yun Gong, Ming Ma, Xia Wang, Yudian Song, Yongxia Wang, Congcheng Chen, Kun Zhang, Xiaoxia Zhou, Guijv Tao, Limin Pan, Qingfeng Xiao, Wenpei Fan, Qinglu Kong, Xiaoyu Li, Xiangqian Fan, Guobin Zhang, Jin Wang, Juan Mou, Meiying Wu, Lisong Chen, Dechao Liu, Shasha Su, and Wenjie Dong. Thanks for your cooperation and help.

There were many professors who provided me their technical support and equipment for my experiments. They are Profs. Jianhua Gao, Yaping Li, Weijun Peng, Yonglian Zhang, Yuchuan Zhou, Zhigang Wang, and Yuanyi Zheng. Thanks for their great help and support. I have also learned a lot from them.

Finally, I want to express the highest appreciation and acknowledgment to my parents. They raised me with their hard work. Meanwhile, I wish to end this part by thanking my dear wife, Lanping Zhang, who was the biggest support for my beloved scientific research. At this time, I want to say I can get everything if I get her full support.

Contents

Chapter 1
Research Background

1.1 Introduction

With the rapid development of modern science and technology, materials science, as one of the most important research frontiers, plays significant roles in promoting human development and social progress. The emergence of each new material will improve the productivity and progress of human society. Especially, polymer materials, metal materials, and inorganic nonmetallic materials, as the most representative three material categories, have found the broad applications in modern science/technology and national economies. Among various material families, porous materials with well-defined mesopores inside the material matrix are a large class of star materials. Their unique structural characteristics, excellent physiochemical properties, and broad applications are always the research frontier in materials science community. According to the definition by International Union of Pure and Applied Chemistry (IUPAC), porous materials can be divided into three categories: microporous materials with the pore size of less than 2 nm, mesoporous materials with the pore size of between 2 and 50 nm, and macroporous materials with the pore size of larger than 50 nm. From the viewpoint of chemical composition, porous materials can be divided into organic, inorganic, and organic/inorganic hybrid porous materials.

As the earliest developed microporous material, zeolite has already achieved the industrial applications in the field of petroleum and chemical catalysis [1, 2]. However, the pore size of zeolite is generally smaller than 2 nm, which severely restricts the diffusion and catalysis of macromolecules within the pores. On this ground, scientists have been committed to fabricate porous materials with well-defined large pores. Until 1992, scientists from Mobil Co. in United States made the significant breakthrough in this research area. Kresge and Beck reported in Nature that ordered mesoporous silica-based materials with the pore size of 1.5–10 nm could be synthesized by a soft surfactant-templating method, which

© Springer-Verlag Berlin Heidelberg 2016
Y. Chen, *Design, Synthesis, Multifunctionalization and Biomedical Applications of Multifunctional Mesoporous Silica-Based Drug Delivery Nanosystems*, Springer Theses, DOI 10.1007/978-3-662-48622-1_1

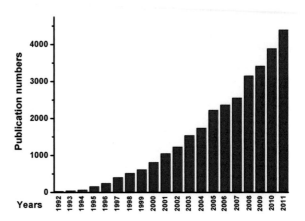

Fig. 1.1 Publications related to mesoporous materials from 1992 to 2011, which was obtained from ISI web of science (*keyword mesoporous*)

substantially broadened the application fields of porous materials [3]. This material family is featured with the large surface area, high pore volume, tunable pore size, controlled morphology, and easily modified inner/outer surface. Importantly, these mesoporous materials make the breakthrough to solve the critical issue of pore size limitation of traditional microporous zeolite. Therefore, this report has attracted the great attentions of science community from physical, chemical, material, and even biological fields.

By the statistic data from Web of Science, it can be found that the number of scientific papers increases substantially every year (Fig. 1.1), indicating that mesoporous materials have been one of the hottest researches since their emergence. Twenty years have gone since the first report in 1992. During this period, mesoporous materials have got very rapid development, from the new synthetic methodology/mechanism to the precise controlling of the crucial structural/compositional parameters. On this ground, various mesoporous material systems have found broad applications in absorption/separation, chemical catalysis, environment treatment, energy, optics, biomedicine, etc., which also show the very promising industrial translation potentials [4, 5].

1.2 Synthetic Methodologies and Structures of Mesoporous Materials

1.2.1 Formation Mechanism of Mesoporous Materials

Templates are generally required to form well-defined mesopores within mesoporous materials. Soft-templating and hard-templating approaches are the two typical and mostly adopted methodologies. The earliest soft-templating approach was based on diverse organic supramolecules as the structural directing agents, such as surfactants, block copolymers, and saline coupling agents [3, 6–7].

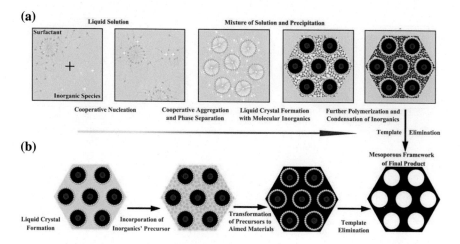

Fig. 1.2 The mechanisms for the synthesis of mesoporous materials: **a** CFM cooperative formation mechanism and **b** LCT liquid-crystal templating mechanism [10]. Reproduced with permission from Ref. [10]. © 2007, American Chemical Society

Comparatively, the hard-templating approach or nanocasting method was based on the infiltration of guest materials within the mesopores of as-synthesized ordered mesoporous silica as the hard template. After further removal of the hard template, well-defined mesoporous structure can be formed [8, 9].

Scientists have proposed several theoretical models to clarify the formation mechanism of the interaction between organic structural directing agents and inorganic species. The representative models include liquid-crystal templating mechanism proposed by Mobil's scientists [3, 6], cooperative formation mechanism by Stucky [11], acid–base pair mechanism by Zhao [12], charge density matching mechanism by Monnier [13], etc. These mechanisms only match specific synthetic systems, among which liquid-crystal templating (LCT) mechanism and cooperative formation mechanism (CFM) are the common principles to explain the formation procedure and mechanism of various mesoporous materials (Fig. 1.2).

1.2.2 Structures of Mesoporous Materials

The microstructure of mesoporous materials is mainly influenced by the interaction and cooperative self-assembly between organic template and inorganic precursor. Controlling the structure of mesoporous materials generally includes the mesopore array and mesopore size. By choosing different surfactants, precursor concentrations, reaction time/temperature, etc., mesoporous materials with abundant microstructures (Fig. 1.3) can be fabricated, such as the mesopores with the geometries of *P6mm, Ia3d, Pm3n, Im3m, Fd3m, Fm3m*, etc., [10].

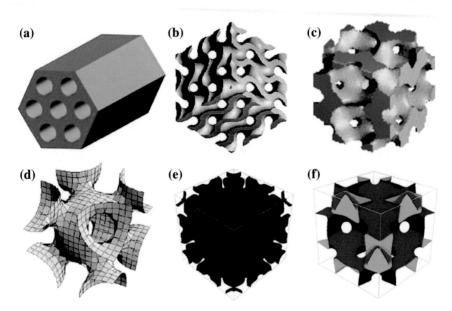

Fig. 1.3 Pore structural models of typical ordered mesoporous materials: **a** *P6mm*, **b** *Ia3d*, **c** *Pm3n*, **d** *Im3m*, **e** *Fd3m* and **f** *Fm3m* [10]. Reproduced with permission from Ref. [10]. © 2007, American Chemical Society

Surfactants are generally employed as the structural directing agents to fabricate mesoporous materials. Therefore, the type and molecular structure of surfactants are important to the formation of mesoporous structures. A widely accepted model was proposed by Israelachvili et al. to predict and explain the formation procedure of mesoporous materials with different structures by surfactants. Surfactant molecular-packing parameter g ($g = V/a_0l$, V: total volume of hydrophobic side chain, a_0: effective area of hydrophobic head, l: dynamic tail length) was introduced for quantitative explanation [14]. By this simple mathematical calculation, it can be predicted which liquid crystal phase could be formed at given condition to form mesoporous structure. Therefore, it can theoretically guide the synthesis of mesoporous material with desirable structures. For example, Huo et al. demonstrated that the g value could effectively control the mesoporous structure in acidic synthetic condition [15]. At $g < 1/3$, SBA-1 with *Pm3n* phase and SBA-2 with *P6_3/mmc* phase were formed. At $1/2 < g < 1/3$, MCM-48 with *Ia3d* phase were generated. At $g \approx 1$, it formed MCM-50 type mesoporous phase. In addition, the intrinsic characteristic of various surfactants also determines the formation of mesoporous materials with diverse mesoporous structures. Abundant mesostructures of mesoporous silica are summarized in Table 1.1.

Table 1.1 The mesostructures of mesoporous silica templated by different SDAs

Space group	Code	Surfactants	References
$P6mm$	MCM41	TMA^+ ($n = 12$–18)	[3, 6]
		$C_{16\text{-}n\text{-}16}$ ($n = 4, 6, 7, 8, 10$)	[15]
		CTAB, $C_{18\text{-}3\text{-}1}$	[16]
		$[(CH_3)_3N^+H_{24}O(C_6H_4)_2OC_{12}H_{24}N^+(CH_3)_3]$ $[2Br^-]$	[16]
		CPBr, $C_nH_{2n+1}N(CH_3)_3$	[17]
	SBA15	P123, P103, P85, P65, B50–1500, Briji97	[18, 19]
	SBA-3	C_nTMA^+ ($n = 14$–18)	[20]
	MSU-H	P123	[21]
	HOM-2	Briji56	[22–27]
$Pm3n$	SBA-1	$C_{16}TEABr$, $H_{33}N(CH_3)(C_2H_5)_2^+$, $C_{18}TMACl$, C_nTAB ($n = 14, 16$), $C_{16\text{-}3\text{-}1}$	[28]
	SBA-6	$C_{16}H_{33}N(C_2H_5)_3^+$	[29]
		$C_{18\text{-}3\text{-}1}$	[24]
$Im3m$	SBA-16	F127	[30]
	FDU-1	B50-6600	[31]
	ST-SBA-16	Brij700	[25]
$Ia3d$	MCM-48	C_nTMA^+(C_nTAB, C_nTACl, C_nTAOH, $n = 14$–20)	[15]
		$C_nTAB^+C_{12}(EO)_m$ ($n = 12, 14, 16, 18$; $m = 3, 4$)	[26]
		$CTAB^+C_{12}NH_2$	[26]
		$CTAB^+C_nH_{2n+1}COONa$ ($n = 11, 13, 15, 17$)	[29]
		$C_{16\text{-}2\text{-}16}$	[15]
	KIT-6	P123	[32]
	FDU-5	P123	[33]
$Pm3m$	SBA-11	Brij56	[30]
	HOM-4	Brij56	[34]
$P6_3/mmc$	HOM-3	Brij56	[22, 23]
	SBA-12	Brij76	[30]
	SBA-2	$C_{12\text{-}3\text{-}1}$, $C_{14\text{-}3\text{-}1}$, $C_{16\text{-}3\text{-}1}$	[15, 35]
		Brij76 ($C_{18}EO_{10}$)	[30]
		F127	[27, 36]
		Omega-hydroxyalkylammouium	[37]
cmm	SBA-8	$[(CH_3)_3N^+H_{24}O(C_6H_4)_2OC_{12}H_{24}N^+(CH_3)_3]$ $[2Br^-]$	[16]
		CTAB	[38]
		P123, Brij58, F127 (film)	[39, 40]
L_3	HOM-6	Brij30 ($C_{12}TO_4$)	[30]
		Brij56	[30]
C_2mm	KSW-2	$C_{16}TMA$	[41]

(continued)

Table 1.1 (continued)

Space group	Code	Surfactants	References
Fd3m	FDU-2	$C_{18-2-3-1}$, $C_{16-2-3-1}$	[42]
	AMS-8	$C_{12}GlyA$	[43]
Fm3m	FDU-12	F127	[44]
	FDU-1	B50-6600	[27]
	KIT-5	F127	[45]
	HOM-10	Brij56	[22]
Disordered	FSM-16	$C_nH_{2n+1}(CH_3)_3N^+Cl^-$, $n = 12-18$	[46, 47]
	HMS	$C_nH_{2n+1}NH_2$, $n = 8-18$	[48, 49]
	KIT-1	HTACl, EDTANa$_4$	[50, 51]
	TUD-1	Triethanolamine	[51]
Chiral	AMS	C14-L-AlaA, C14-L-AlaS	[52]
Vescile	MSU-G	$C_nH_{2n+1}NH(CH_2)_2NH_2$	[53, 54]
Foam	MCF	P123, TMB	[42]
Hollow	HMSNs	CTAB, $C_{18}TMS$	[55−57]

1.3 Biomedical Applications of Mesoporous Materials

The initial aim of synthesizing mesoporous materials was to realize the catalytic reaction of macromolecules by controlling the mesopore sizes. Therefore, the catalytic applications of mesoporous materials as the catalysts develop very fast. Various mesoporous material systems have been synthesized, including silica-based and non-silica-based mesoporous materials, which present high catalytic activities [4]. In addition, the large surface area, high pore volume and tunable pore size of mesopores endow mesoporous materials with high performance in environment treatment, such as absorption of heavy metal ions, CO_2 absorption at room temperature and catalytic transition/absorption of toxic NOx gases [58−60]. Carbon-based mesoporous materials have found the applications in electrochemical fields, such as PEMFC, lithium-ion battery, supercapacitors, etc., [61]. Recently, mesoporous materials show the high performance in biomedicine, such as drug encapsulation/delivery/controlled release, molecular imaging, tissue engineering, enzyme/protein immobilization, etc. For example, hollow mesoporous spheres synthesized by our research group exhibited high drug-loading capacity, targeted drug transportation and multimode diagnostic imaging performance [62, 63].

Nanobiotechnology has become a hot research frontier relating to the multidisciplinary of material science, chemistry, biotechnology, and biomedicine because of its high application potentials in human health/biomedicine and corresponding large economic benefits. With the development of science/technology and high assumption of human health, it is highly desirable to develop new diagnostic and therapeutic approaches to realize the early diagnosis of diseases and efficient therapy of confirmed diseases with high performance and mitigated side effects.

Fig. 1.4 Scheme of a nanotheranostic system for tumor diagnosis and therapy based on mesoporous silica

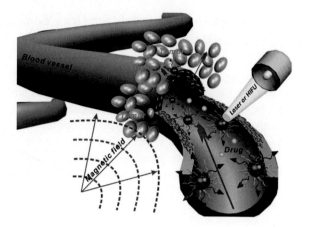

To achieve this aim, the precise diagnosis of specific diseases and targeted drug delivery is of high significance (Fig. 1.4). Various drug delivery nanosystems have been synthesized based on nanobiotechnology and nano-synthetic chemistry, including organic, inorganic, and organic/inorganic material nanosystems. The organic carriers suffer from the drawbacks of low thermal/chemical stability and low drug-loading capacity. The drugs will be released explosively upon the disintegration of the organic carriers, which cannot achieve the goals of sustained drug releasing and continuous therapy. Comparatively, inorganic carriers are featured with high chemical/thermal stability, high drug-loading capacity, and easy surface functionalization, showing the extensive application prospects in nanobiotechnology.

Ordered mesoporous materials possess large surface area, high pore volume, well-defined mesoporous structure, easily modified inner/outer surface, and excellent chemical/thermal stability. These characteristics indicate that mesoporous materials can act as excellent drug delivery systems (designated as DDSs). Since the first report on the drug-loading and sustained release from MCM-41-type mesoporous silica on 2001 [64], mesoporous materials as the drug carriers have attracted great attention of scientists over the world [65]. Mesoporous silica nanoparticles (designated as MSNs) with different nanostructures and morphologies have been fabricated as the drug delivery nanosystem. Meanwhile, various drugs, including antiphlogistic drugs, hydrophilic/hydrophobic anticancer drugs, antibacterial drugs, genes, anti-hepatic fibrosis drugs, have been encapsulated and delivered by using mesoporous materials as the drug delivery carrier. Recently, the functional design and biological evaluation of mesoporous materials have become one of the research frontiers. For biological safety, the evaluations of mesoporous silica have developed from initial in vitro cell level to systematic in vivo assessments, including cytotoxicities, blood compatibility, biodegradation, biodistribution, excretion, etc. The preliminary pharmacokinetics and pharmacodynamics were also revealed on several mice tumor xenografts.

1.3.1 Mesoporous Materials for Drug Loading and Sustained Release

The early report on the drug delivery by mesoporous materials was focused on the sustained release of drugs based on the porous structure of mesoporous materials, from the earliest MCM41-type mesoporous silica reported by Vallet-Regí to further MCM-48 and SBA15-type mesoporous silica materials [64, 65]. Some crucial parameters, such as pore size, surface area, pore volume, pore symmetry, and surface status were found to be important on the encapsulation and release of drugs from mesopores. Because of the steric effect, the drug-loading capacity of mesoporous materials with small mesopores is lower than that of mesoporous materials with large mesopores. For example, the loading capacity of bovine serum albumin within SBA15 increased from 15 to 27 % after the enlargement of mesopores from initial 8.2 to 11.4 nm. In addition, the drug-releasing rate decreased when the pore size of MCM-41 was reduced [66]. The mesopore structure could also influence the drug encapsulation and subsequent releasing, especially for the penetration and geometry of mesopores. The drug-releasing rate from penetrating mesopores is faster than that of non-penetrating mesopores. For example, SBA-1 with three-dimensional penetrating mesopores showed faster drug-releasing rate compared to SBA-3 with non-penetrating mesopores, though they had the similar pore size and surface area. The change of surface area and pore volume causes the variations of drug-loading amount. The surface status also has a determining influence to the diffusion of drug molecules into the mesopores, thus it leads to controllable drug-loading capacity and releasing behavior.

In addition to traditional mesoporous silica, such as MCM-41, MCM-48, and SBA15, hollow mesoporous silica nanoparticles (designated as HMSNs) with large hollow cavity have attracted the extensive attention. The large hollow interior of HMSNs leaves much more room for drug molecules, thus their drug-loading capacity is high. The well-defined mesoporous structure provides the diffusion paths for drug molecules. The high drug-loading capacity also means that less carrier will be used at the same drug dose. This merit can reduce the introduction and deposition of foreign matters within the body, thus the biocompatibility is high. Our research group found that the IBU-loading amount within HMSNs was 744.5 mg/g, much higher than MCM-41 type MSNs (358.6 mg/g). Because of the similar surface area and pore volume, the double increased drug-loading amount was attributed to the large hollow interior of HMSN [67]. Furthermore, our group employed Fe_3O_4 nanoparticles as the hard template to fabricate HMSNs with different morphologies, which also showed the high drug-loading capacity [55].

1.3.2 Mesoporous Materials for Controlled Drug Releasing

It is highly desirable to design and fabricate DDSs with precisely controlled drug-releasing behavior, which can improve the therapeutic efficiency and mitigate the side effects of drugs. Upon arriving at the targeted lesion site, these DDSs release the loaded drugs by internal or external triggers [68, 69]. The pre-releasing and even zero-releasing can be realized by these DDSs. For mesoporous materials, a large amount of macromolecules or nanoparticles have been designed as the nano-valves to seal the drugs within the mesopores. Upon internal/external triggering, these nanovalves can be opened to release the drugs. The purpose of controlled drug releasing can be realized via this protocol. Based on MSNs, different con-trolled drug-releasing patterns have been explored, such as pH, redox, tempera-ture, ultrasound, enzyme, light, antigen–antibody reaction, glucose, etc.

For instance, pH-responsive drug releasing is based on the pH varia-tions between tumor (pH $\approx$ 6.5) and normal tissue (pH $\approx$ 7.4). In addition, the endosomes and lysosomes of cells present more acidic microenvironment (ca. 5.0–5.5) [70–72]. Our group reported for the first time that a unique type of mesoporous silica-based pH-responsive DDSs could be constructed by surface modification with polyelectrolyte [68]. As shown in Fig. 1.5a–f, the surface of HMSNs was coated by a layer of polyelectrolyte (PAH and PSS), which could expand and contract under different pH environment, leading to the responsive drug releasing. Importantly, this polyelectrolyte layer was also responsive to the ion strength for responsive drug releasing. Recently, MSNs-based controlled drug releasing was realized in vivo. Bhatia et al. coated a bio-responsive PEG layer onto the surface of MSNs [69]. Anticancer drug doxorubicin could be released within the tumor tissue by the abundant protease, causing the death of tumor cells. Other representative MSNs-based controlled drug-releasing patterns are summa-rized in Table 1.2.

1.3.3 Mesoporous Materials for Photodynamic Therapy

Surgery, radiotherapy, and chemotherapy are the three main treatment approaches for tumor. These therapeutic modalities unavoidably cause the damage and death of normal cells when they remove and kill the cancer cells, leading to serious side effects and complications. The development of new therapeutic modality with higher efficiency and lower side effects is highly desirable. As a new therapeu-tic modality developed in 1970s, photodynamic therapy is a promising technology for clinical cancer treatment. After the injection of photosensitizers, these photo-responsive photosensitizer molecules can passively or positively target into tumor tissue. After the irradiation by light at specific wavelength, the photosensitizers can produce highly active singlet oxygen, which is highly toxic to induce the death of cancer cells. Compared to other therapeutic modalities, photodynamic therapy directly focuses the laser onto the lesion part and triggers the releasing of singlet oxygen to kill the cancer cell. The unexposed tissue to light will not be harmed by toxic singlet oxygen. Thus, the side effects are substantially mitigated.

Because the mesopores channel facilitates the high loading of guest molecules, MSNs are regarded as the DDSs to encapsulate and transfer the photosensitizers

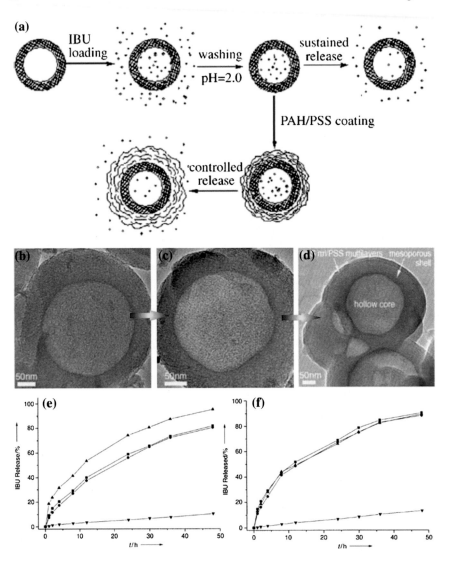

Fig. 1.5 a Schematic illustration of synthetic strategy for pH-responsive DDSs based on polyelectrolyte multilayers coating; TEM images of HMSNs (**b**), IBU-HMSNs (**c**) and polyelectrolyte-coated IBU-HMSNs (**d**); pH− (**e**) and ion strength-responsive (**f**) ibuprofen (IBU) release from the polyelectrolyte-coated IBU-HMSNs; Reproduced with permission from Ref. [68]. © 2005, WILEY-VCH Verlag GmbH & Co. KGaA, Weinheim

for photodynamic therapy. Mou et al. grafted photosensitizer protoporphyrin (PpIX-MSNs) into the mesopores of MSNs for photodynamic therapy. By the external laser irradiation at the wavelength of 514 nm, the singlet oxygen was produced to kill HeLa cancer cells (Fig. 1.6) [103]. Li et al. further coated a phospholipid layer onto the surface of MSNs to improve their capability for intracellular

Table 1.2 Representative stimuli-responsive DDSs based on MSNs

MSNs type	Surface modification and nanovalves	Triggers	Guest molecules	References
MCM-41	Coumarin	Light	Cholestane	[73]
MCM-41	Au NPs	Light	Palitaxel	[74]
MCM-41	Poly(NIPAMNBAE)	Light	Fluorescein	[75]
MCM-41	Azobenzene derivatives	Light	Rhodamine B	[76]
MCM-41	Mercaptopropyl	Light	Sulforhodamine 101 and [Ru(bpy)$_2$(PPh$_3$)Cl]Cl	[77]
MCM-41	Coumarin	Light	Chlorambucil	[78]
MCM-41	Au NPs	pH, light	Safranine O	[79]
SBA-15	PDDA	pH	Vancomycin	[80]
MCM-41	PEI/CD	pH	Calcein	[81]
Hollow MSNs	Polyelectrolyte	pH	Ibuprofen	[68]
MCM-41	PDEAEMA	pH	Rhodamine B	[82]
MCM-41	Hydrazone bonds	pH	Doxorubicin	[83]
MCM-41	DNA	pH	Rhodamine B	[84]
MCM-41	PMV	pH	Ibuprofen	[85]
MCM-41	Poly(acrylic acid)	pH	Fluorescein	[86]
MCM-41	Fe$_3$O$_4$ NPs	Redox	Fluorescein	[87]
MCM-41	CdS NPs	Redox	Vancomycin & ATP	[88]
MCM-41	Poly(N-acryloxysuccimide)	Redox	Rhodamine B	[89]
MCM-41	Lactose	Enzyme	[Ru(bipy)$_3$]Cl$_2$	[90]
MCM-41	Saccharide	Enzyme	[Ru(bipy)$_3$]Cl$_2$ and doxorubicin	[91]
MCM-41	Peptide sequence	Enzyme	[Ru(bipy)$_3$]Cl$_2$	[92]
MCM-41	[2]rotaxanes	Enzyme	Rhodamine B	[93]
MCM-41	Cyclodextrin	Enzyme	Calcein	[94]
MCM-41	Avidin	Enzyme	Fluorescein	[95]
MCM-41	PNIPAM	Temperature	Fluorescein	[96]
Fe$_3$O$_4$@mSiO$_2$	PNIPAM	Temperature	ZnPcS$_4$	[97]
Magnetic SBA-15	PNIPAM	Temperature	Gentamicin	[98]
MCM-41	Antibody	Antigen–antibody reaction	[Ru(bipy)$_3$]Cl$_2$	[99]
MCM-41	G-ins proteins	Glucose	Insulin and cyclic AMP	[100]
MCM-41	Poly(dimethylsiloxane)	Ultrasound	Ibuprofen	[101]
MCM-41	DNA	DNA degradation	Rhodamine B	[102]

Fig. 1.6 Schematic
illustration of cell apoptosis
by photosensitizer-loaded
MSNs under the light
irradiation

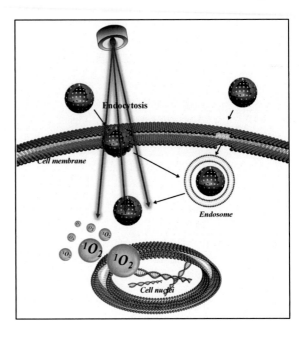

transport of photosensitizer [104]. They also successfully demonstrated that the
produced singlet oxygen by laser irradiation caused the high cytotoxicity to cancer
cells.

1.3.4 Mesoporous Materials for Synergistic Therapy

During the chemotherapeutic process, the frequent drug administration causes
the multidrug resistance (MDR) of cancer cells. Higher drug doses are required
to achieve the desirable therapeutic outcome. However, the excessive drug utiliza-
tion would cause severe side effects. Recently developed multidrug combination
can effectively suppress the MDR of cancer cells and enhance the therapeutic efficiency of single drugs [105].

MSNs provide the promising platform for co-loading and co-delivery of mul-
tidrugs. They show the unique merits for the co-delivery of small drug molecules
and large therapeutic macromolecules. On the one hand, the large surface area
and high pore volume of MSNs can be used as the reservoir for small molecules.
On the other hand, the controlled surface chemical property makes the anchoring of macromolecules possible, such as DNA and siRNA. Chen et al. encapsulated doxorubicin (DOX) into the mesopores, and employed dendrimer to anchor
siRNA to inhibit the expression of Bcl-2 (Fig. 1.7a) [106]. The MDR of A2780/
AD cancer cells was efficiently suppressed by this co-delivery strategy. The
introduction of BCl-2-siRNA silenced the expression of Bcl-2-mRNA, thus the

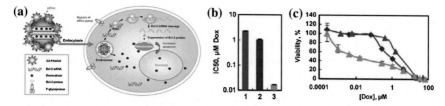

Fig. 1.7 a Schematic illustration of co-delivering DOX and Bcl-2-targeted siRNA simultaneously based on MSNs for enhanced chemotherapy efficacy; IC_{50} (**b**) of, and cell viability curves (**c**) after co-incubation with (*1*) free DOX (*blue*), (*2*) MSNs-DOX-G2 (*red*) and (*3*) MSNs-DOX-G2/siRNA (*green*). Reproduced with permission from Ref. [106]. © 2009, WILEY-VCH Verlag GmbH & Co. KGaA, Weinheim

expression of Bcl-2 protein was inhibited. Finally, the non-pumping type DOX resistance was suppressed and the cytotoxicity of DOX against cancer cells was enhanced (Fig. 1.7b–d). Similarly, Lin et al. encapsulated DOX into the mesopores of MSNs, and grafted PEI on the surface to absorb siRNA by electrostatic interaction to inhibit the expression of P-gp [107]. Based on this co-delivery strategy, the pumping-related MDR of KB-V1 cancer cells was suppressed and the therapeutic efficiency of DOX was improved.

Our group also achieved the important progress on multidrug-based synergistic therapy. Dr. He et al. employed micelles formed by surfactants (C_{16}TAB) to load DOX during the synthetic procedure of MSNs [108]. Different from traditional method to remove the surfactants by either calcination or extraction, C_{16}TAB molecules were kept within the mesopores to act as the chemotherapeutic sensitizer to suppress the MDR of MCF-7/ADR cancer cells, which could also enhance the cytotoxicity of DOX against cancer cells.

1.3.5 MSNs for Targeted Drug Delivery

For DDSs, the most important issue is to realize the targeted delivery. Targeted drug delivery can directly deliver the therapeutic agents into cancer cells and release them right at the targeted site. Therefore, targeted drug delivery is featured with high sensitivity and specificity. For tumor chemotherapy, the high permeability of tumor blood vessels is generally regarded and used as the enhanced permeability retention (EPR) effect to realize passive targeted drug delivery. However, the efficiency of such a passive targeting is relatively low, which is difficult to achieve the high therapeutic modality. Active targeting is featured with high efficiency, which is generally realized by modifying the surface of DDSs with targeting molecules, antibodies, aptamers, etc. These surface-modified targeting modules can effectively recognize the overexpressed molecules, factors, or antigens on the surface of cancer cells to enhance the accumulation of DDSs within tumor tissue. Active targeting is much more efficient than passive targeting, showing high application potentials.

Two typical strategies have been developed to endow MSNs with targeting function: One is targeting to the cell membrane and the other is targeting to the intracellular organelles. Folic acid receptor (FA) is overexpressed on the membrane of many cancer cells, which is generally regarded as the targeting site for drug delivery. Rohsenholm et al. grafted FA onto the surface of MSNs for FA receptor targeting. The results showed that FA-overexpressed cancer cells had nearly fivefold increase in the uptake amount of MSNs compared to non-targeted cancer cells (Fig. 1.8a–g) [109]. Anti-HER2/neu mAb antibody was grafted onto the surface of MSNs to target Her2-overexpressed breast cancer cells. By TEM observation, it was found that antibody-grafted MSNs were endocytosized into cancer cells by using acceptor-mediated path [111]. DNA aptamer was modified onto the surface of polyelectrolyte-coated MSNS for concurrent cell targeting and stimuli-responsive drug releasing [112]. Our group modified the surface of MSNs by hyaluronic acid (HA) for targeting CD44-overexpressed HeLa cells [113]. The HA modification also improved the dispersity and stability of MSNs in physiological conditions.

Recently, our group designed TAT-modified MSNs for targeting the nucleus of cancer cells [110]. The presence of TAT could endow MSNs with the specific capability to enter the nucleus through nuclear pore. In addition, the particle size also determines the possibility of MSNs-TAT entering the nucleus of cells. Figure 1.8h–m shows the intra-nuclear drug delivery by MSNs-TAT with the particle size of 25–50 nm. Importantly, intra-nuclear drug delivery could significantly enhance the cytotoxicities of DOX for killing the cancer cells.

Although the preliminary targeting strategies of MSNs can enhance the drug accumulation within cancer cells and bring with the improved therapeutic efficiency, the complex physiological environment of body makes the efficient in vivo targeting difficult. In vivo targeted drug delivery requires stricter control on the key structural/compositional parameters of MSNs, such as particle size, surface status, surface charge, dispersity, and stability, which play the determining role for successful in vivo targeting. On this ground, the precise control of these parameters should be further achieved to guarantee the possible efficient in vivo targeted drug delivery.

1.3.6 Mesoporous Materials for Theranostic Applications

The development of nano-synthetic chemistry provides the theoretical and methodological base for the multifunctionalization of MSNs, by which unique MSNs-based theranostic nanosystems can be fabricated with concurrent diagnostic and therapeutic functions. The merits of these MSNs-based theranostic carriers are their capability to find the lesion tissue before the administration. In addition, they can also realize the in situ monitoring of therapeutic process and provide the information of the therapeutic outcome, facilitating the further adjusting of the treatment protocol. Because of the high performance and extensive application,

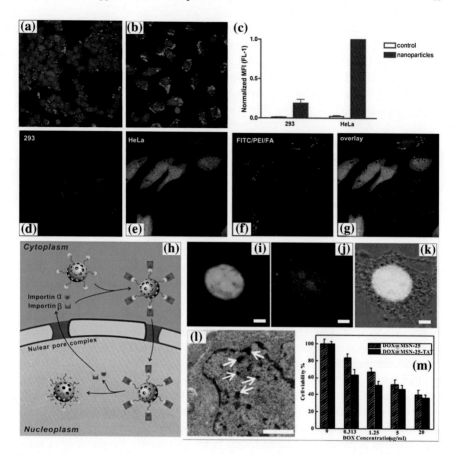

Fig. 1.8 The in vitro evaluation of the targeting efficiency of folic acid modified MSNs using 293 cells (**a**, expressing low-level folate receptors) and HeLa cells (**b**, expressing high-level folate receptors) using confocal microscopy (**a–b** and **d–g**) and flow cytometry (**c**, meal fluorescence intensity of FITC in cells). In addition, HeLa and 293 cells were labeled with *blue* CMAC (**e**) and CellTracker *Red* (**d**), respectively, to directly observe the targeting efficiency of folic acid modified MSNs (**f** and **g**); Reproduced with permission from Ref. [109]. © 2009, American Chemical Society. **h** Schematic illustration of TAT peptide-conjugated MSNs (MSNs-TAT) for intra-nucleus drug delivery; (**i–k**) CLSM images of nucleus-accumulation of MSNs-TAT (**i** DAPI, **j** *green* fluorescence for MSNs-TAT and **k** overlapped image) within HeLa cells; **l** Bio-TEM image of HeLa cells after the co-incubation with MSNs-TAT; **m** Cell viabilities of HeLa cells after the co-incubation with DOX@MSNs and DOX@MSNs-TAT (25 nm). Reproduced with permission from Ref. [110]. © 2012, American Chemical Society

theranostic nanomedicine has become one of the hottest research frontiers in bio-medicine. Compared to traditional mesoporous SiO_2-based DDSs, such a multi-functionalization design can endow the carrier with specific function based on the practical clinical requirements. The most representative feature of mesoporous theranostic particles is their capability of concurrent diagnostic imaging and therapy. For instance, magnetic MSNs not only can act as the contrast agents of T_2-weighted MR imaging, but also can be used for magnetic field-guided targeted drug delivery and hyperthermia. Fluorescent MSNs can label the cancer cells, monitor the drug release, and can be used in vivo fluorescent imaging. Furthermore, the elaborate design at nanoscale can integrate more functions into one matrix (MSNs) to endow the carrier with the functions of multimodality diagnostic imaging and efficient drug delivery.

1.3.6.1 Magnetic Resonance Imaging (MRI)

Magnetic mesoporous SiO_2 materials are the earliest and the most explored composite material systems for biomedical applications [63, 114−116]. The magnetic functionalization of MSNs can play the roles of magnetic targeting, magnetic hyperthermia and T_2-weighted MR imaging. Although magnetic targeting and magnetic hyperthermia show the promising clinical translation to benefit the patients, their research is relatively rare because of the technical limitation [116]. Comparatively, magnetic MSNs are mostly explored as the mature T_2-weighted MRI contrast agents.

Two typical approaches have been developed to integrate the magnetic module into MSNs (Fig. 1.9). On the one hand, the surface of magnetic nanoparticles can be coated by a mesoporous silica layer by sol-gel process. On the other hand, magnetic nanoparticles can be anchored onto the surface of mesoporous silica by covalent bonds. The coating procedure generally employs the surfactants or saline coupling agents as the structural directing agents. Our group for the first time synthesized $Fe_3O_4@SiO_2@mSiO_2$ composite nanoparticles by using $C_{18}TMS$ as the pore-making agent. After loading IBU into the mesopores, they showed sustained drug-releasing behavior in simulated body fluid. Importantly, the presence of magnetic core could manipulate the nanoparticles by external magnetic field [117]. Zhao et al. also employed layer-by-layer coating procedure to successfully fabricate $Fe_3O_4@SiO_2@mSiO_2$ magnetic composite nanoparticles by using $C_{16}TAB$ as the structural directing agent [118]. Hyeon et al. successfully fabricated magnetic $Fe_3O_4@mSiO_2$ with the particle size of less than 100 nm [115, 119]. Hydrophobic Fe_3O_4 nanoparticles were initially synthesized, followed by phase transformation from organic medium into aqueous solution assisted by amphiphilic $C_{16}TAB$ surfactant. After further introduction of silica source, a uniform mesoporous silica layer was formed onto the surface of hydrophobic Fe_3O_4 nanoparticles. $C_{16}TAB$ acted not only as the phase-transferring agent, but also as the structural directing agent. After further surface PEGylation, these magnetic mesoporous nanoparticles could accumulate into tumor tissues by EPR effect. The magnetic core was used as the T_2-weighted MRI contrast agents with r_2 value of 245 mM^{-1} s^{-1}. The tumors could also be clearly observed by MR imaging after 24 h intravenous injection of $Fe_3O_4@mSiO_2$ nanoparticles.

Anchoring magnetic nanoparticles onto the surface of MSNs is another efficient approach to fabricate magnetic mesoporous composite nanoparticles. The merits of this method include the easy controlling of the loading amount of

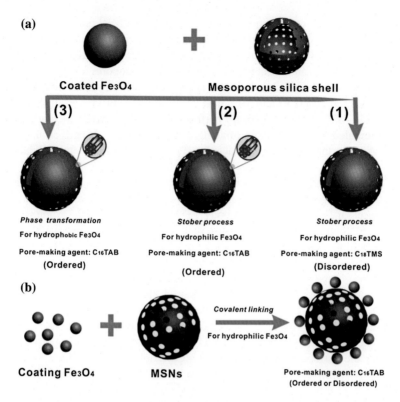

Fig. 1.9 Summarization of the general synthetic strategies for magnetic mesoporous silica-based composite nanoparticles, including coating mesoporous silica shell onto the surface of Fe_3O_4 nanoparticles (**a**, Coated Fe_3O_4) and binding Fe_3O_4 NPs onto the surface of MSNs (**b**, Coating Fe_3O_4)

magnetic nanoparticles and the whole particle size. Hyeon et al. anchored magnetic nanoparticles onto the surface of dye-doped MSNs (designated as mSiO$_2$@Fe$_3$O$_4$) for concurrent T_2-weighted MR imaging and DOX delivery [120]. The results presented that the tumor of mice was clearly observed after the intravenous administration of mSiO$_2$@Fe$_3$O$_4$ composite nanoparticles. In addition, the delivery of DOX significantly induced the death of cancer cells. Magnetic nanoparticles could also act as the nanovalves to seal the drug within the mesopores by pH-reversible covalent bonds for controlled drug releasing [121].

The accessibility of paramagnetic centers to water molecules determines the performance of T_1-weighted MR imaging [122−124]. Based on this design principle, the dispersity of paramagnetic centers should be enhanced to increase the interaction chances between paramagnetic centers and water molecules. Mesoporous materials are featured with tunable mesoporous size, large surface area, and high pore volume, thus they are one of the most desirable carriers to disperse the paramagnetic centers [10].

Gd-based chelates are the most adopted T_1-weighted MRI contrast agent [122, 123]. By dispersion of Gd-based paramagnetic centers into the mesopores, it was expected that a new type high performance T_1-weighted MRI contrast agents could be obtained. Lin et al. modified the inner mesopores of MCM-41 type MSNs by Gd–Si-DTTA [124]. In vitro result showed that r_1 could reach as high as 28.8 mM^{-1} s^{-1} (3.0 T) and 10.2 mM^{-1} s^{-1} (9.4 T). In vivo evaluation demonstrated Gd-MSNs could effectively perform T_1-weighted MRI vascular imaging and T_2-weighted MRI soft tissue imaging at the high dose. Huang et al. grafted Gd-DTPA onto the mesopore surface for T_1-weighted MRI stem cell labeling [125].

Although Gd-based MRI-T_1 contrast agents have got the extensive clinical application, their potential toxicity is the critical issue to be solved because Gd is not the necessary element in human body. FDA has warned that the administration of Gd-based contrast agents might cause nephrogenic systemic fibrosis, hypersensitivity reactions and nephrogenic fibrosing dermopathy [126−128]. Therefore, searching for alternative new MRI-T_1 contrast agents has attracted great research attention. Mn-based MRI-T_1 contrast agents are very promising to substitute Gd-based agents, because Mn(II) has five unpaired electrons, showing high relaxation time [129−131]. Importantly, Mn element is the indispensable rare element of body and it involves the body's metabolism. Mn element can also be controlled by body homeostasis. On this ground, Hyeon et al. coated a mesoporous silica layer onto the surface of hollow MnO nanoparticles for T_1-weighted MRI stem cell tracking [132]. The r_1 value was only 0.99 mM^{-1} s^{-1}, which was due to the shielding effect of paramagnetic centers of MnO nanoparticles from water molecules by mesoporous silica coating. Chou et al. further systematically investigated the MRI-T_1 performance of solid MnO, hollow MnO, solid MnO@mSiO$_2$ and hollow MnO@mSiO$_2$, and employed mesopores to load Ir complex as the photosensitizer for photodynamic therapy [130]. Although mesopores facilitate the diffusion of water molecules and enhance the interaction chances between water molecules and Mn paramagnetic centers, the MRI-T_1 performance of solid MnO ($r_1 = 0.17$ mM^{-1} s^{-1}), hollow MnO ($r_1 = 0.92$ mM^{-1} s^{-1}), solid MnO@mSiO$_2$ ($r_1 = 0.16$ mM^{-1} s^{-1}), and hollow MnO@mSiO$_2$ ($r_1 = 0.2$ mM^{-1} s^{-1}) was still much lower than clinical Gd-based contrast agents. It is highly desirable to develop new Mn-based contrast agents with high performance for MR imaging, which is expected to be realized by rational design and synthesis of nanoparticulate systems with optimized nanostructures and compositions.

1.3.6.2 Fluorescent Imaging

Each diagnostic imaging modality has the advantage and limitation. For instance, the spatial resolution of MRI is high, but its sensitivity is low. Fluorescent imaging is featured with low cost, high sensitivity, high efficiency, and in situ drug-releasing observation, showing high clinical application for diagnostic imaging. Based on the development of nano-synthetic chemistry, various fluorescent biomaterials with optimized composition, structure, and fluorescent property have been fabricated, such as organic fluorescein, quantum dots, upconversion nanocrystals, silicon quantum dots, carbon nanodots, etc., [136—142]. Functionalization of MSNs with fluorescent module can render the carrier with the capability of concurrent drug delivery and fluorescent imaging. For organic fluorescein, Lo et al. used FDA-approved near-infrared organic fluorescein—indocyanine green to be absorbed onto trimethylammonium-modified mesopores of MSNs via electrostatic interaction—which was further used as the near-infrared contrast agents for fluorescent imaging [143]. However, the quantum efficiency and photostability of organic fluorescein are low. Comparatively, semiconductor quantum dots are featured with tunable fluorescent emission, wide excitation spectrum, high quantum yield and photostability, showing the extensive applications in cell labeling and in vivo fluorescent imaging. For example, Pan et al. encapsulated CdSe/ZnS quantum dots into the inner core of MSNs for the efficient labeling and imaging of cancer cells [144]. It is noted that Cd-containing quantum dots have relatively high potential toxicity, limiting their further clinical translations.

In addition, rare earth-doped nano-biomaterials can emit the fluorescence from ultraviolet to near-infrared by doping different rare earth ions under 980 nm laser excitation. Compared to semiconductor quantum dots, rare earth-doped upconversion materials do not involve toxic Cd element, showing higher biocompatibility. Qian et al. synthesized $NaYF_4:Yb/Er@SiO_2@mSiO_2$ nanoparticles for the encapsulation of zinc phthalocyanine photosensitizer. Under the 980 nm laser excitation, $NaYF_4:Yb/Er$ was used for cell labeling and fluorescent imaging. In addition, the emission of visible light activated the loaded photosensitizer to generate toxic singlet oxygen and kill the cancer cells [145]. Importantly, the excitation and emission wavelength of rare earth-doped fluorescent nanoparticles can be precisely adjusted by selecting different co-doped ions. In this regard, fluorescent nanoparticles with concurrent near-infrared excitation and near-infrared emission can be fabricated, which is of high significance for in vivo fluorescent imaging because of the improved tissue-penetrating depth and reduced spontaneous fluorescence interference. Therefore, rare earth-doped fluorescent mesoporous theranostic nanosystems show broad applications in fluorescent imaging.

Although upconversion fluorescent nanoparticles are more biocompatible than Cd-based semiconductor quantum dots, the rare earth elements are not the essential elements within the body. The excessive intake might also bring with the potential toxicity issue. Comparatively, silicon quantum dots only contain the silica element, thus their biocompatibility and biosafety are much higher. The integration of silicon quantum dots with MSNs can also realize concurrent fluorescent imaging and drug delivery, but their biocompatibility is improved compared to other fluorescent mesoporous nanosystems.

Our group recently developed a bottom-up self-assembly approach to introduce triethoxysilane as the silicon source during the synthetic procedure for fabricating MSNs (Fig. 1.10). Large amounts of oxygen vacancies were generated by high temperature treatment and dehydrogenation. Fluorescent property was rendered by oxygen deficiency (Fig. 1.10h) [134]. The fluorescent spectrum presented that the

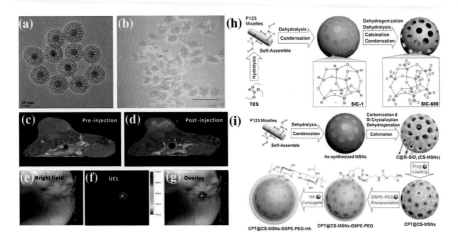

Fig. 1.10 **a** TEM image of NaYF$_4$:Tm/Yb/Gd@mSiO$_2$ nanocomposite particles; **b** Confocal fluorescent images MCF-7 cells after co-incubation with NaYF$_4$:Tm/Yb/Gd@mSiO$_2$ NPs; In vivo T$_1$-weighted MRI (**c** and **d**) and upconversion luminescence imaging (**e, f,** and **g**) of tumor before (**c** and **e**) and after (**d, f,** and **g**) the administration of NaYF$_4$:Tm/Yb/Gd@m SiO$_2$ NPs; Reproduced with permission from Ref. [133]. © 2012, WILEY-VCH Verlag GmbH & Co. KGaA, Weinheim. **h** Schematic illustration for the preparation of oxygen-deficient fluorescent MSNs and **i** carbon-containing fluorescent MSNs. (**h**) Reproduced with permission from Ref. [134]. © 2012, The Royal Society of Chemistry. (**i**) Reproduced with permission from Ref. [135]. © 2012, Elsevier

emission spectrum was wide, and the fluorescent intensity was enhanced by the post-calcination treatment. These fluorescent MSNs were further used for cancer cell labeling and DOX intracellular delivery. After further introduction of hydrophobic carbon component by in situ carbonization approach (Fig. 1.10j), the loading capacity of the carrier for hydrophobic anticancer agents was enhanced [135]. Although the biosafety of silicon quantum dots is high, their fluorescent performance is still much lower compared to traditional semiconductor quantum dots and upconversion nanocrystals. On this ground, the following research should be focused on the improvement of their fluorescent performance to meet the requirement of in vivo fluorescent imaging.

1.3.6.3 Multi-modality Diagnostic Imaging

By the elaborate design at nanoscale, more functional modules can be integrated into MSNs for multimodality diagnostic imaging. For instance, fluorescent imaging could be endowed into magnetic MSNs for concurrent MR imaging and fluorescent imaging. During the fabrication of magnetic/fluorescent dual functional MSNs, magnetic Fe$_3$O$_4$ and fluorescent CdSe/ZnS was concurrently coated by a mesoporous silica layer [119]. In addition, Nd^{3+} and Yb^{3+} co-doped organic chelates were introduced into the mesopores of Fe$_3$O$_4$@mSiO$_2$ for dual diagnostic imaging [146]. The surface of $Fe_3O_4@mSiO_2$ was also coated by quantum dots for multifunctionalization [147].

Furthermore, our group successfully coated a uniform mesoporous silica layer onto the surface of $NaYF_4$:Tm/Yb/Gd nanoparticles ($NaYF_4$:Tm/Yb/Gd@mSiO_2) [133]. $NaYF_4$:Tm/Yb/Gd core presented upconversion fluorescence and T_1-weighted MR imaging capability because of the presence of Gd. Therefore, $NaYF_4$:Tm/Yb/ Gd@mSiO_2 nanoparticles acted as the dual fluorescent/MR imaging contrast agents (Fig. 1.10a–g). The mesoporous silica shell was used for the encapsulation and delivery of therapeutic agents. In vitro and in vivo evaluations showed that $NaYF_4$:Tm/ Yb/Gd@mSiO_2 could be used for cancer cell labeling/in vivo fluorescent imaging and T_1-weighted MR imaging ($r_1 = 3.07$ mM^{-1} s^{-1}). Au nanorods were assembled onto the surface of $Fe_3O_4@SiO_2@mSiO_2$ nanoparticles for concurrent near-infrared imaging, dark-field light cell labeling, MR imaging and chemo/thermal synergistic therapy [148]. Under the 808 nm laser excitation, these composite nanosystems absorbed the near-infrared laser for photothermal therapy. The synergistic therapeutic efficiency was much higher than single therapeutic modality assisted by Au-decorated $Fe_3O_4@SiO_2@mSiO_2$ nanoparticles.

1.4 The Development Trends of Mesoporous Materials

The research on mesoporous materials has developed for more than 20 years. Large amounts of researches have shown that the precise controlling of the morphology, structure, and composition of mesoporous materials can render them with unique properties and high performance in broad applications. However, their large-scale preparation and industrial applications are still very rare, which is mainly attributed to the high cost and poor stability of mesoporous materials. On this ground, it is necessary to develop new simple, economic, environment-friendly methodologies to synthesize mesoporous materials with desirable key parameters. In addition, the formation mechanism of mesoporous materials has not been fully revealed, which should be further verified and corrected by more advanced characterization methods. The most important issue is to fabricate mesoporous materials with more stable structures to meet the requirements of large-scale industrial applications. In biomedicine, there is an urgent need for the rigorous, systematic, and accurate evaluations for the biological effects and biosafety of various mesoporous biomaterials.

1.5 Significance of this Thesis

Based on the development of materials science and biomedicine, a growing number of medical problems can be solved by nanobiotechnology, which also promotes the progress of nano-synthetic chemistry and materials science. It is one of the leading trends to design, synthesis and biomedical applications of diverse biomaterials for solving the critical issues in clinic. Mesoporous biomaterials are featured with unique size effect, quantum effect, large surface area, chemical activity, and biological behavior, showing high application potentials in the early diagnosis and efficient therapy of serious diseases.

Elaborate design and integration of various functional molecules, organic gorups, and nanoparticles with mesoporous silica can meet the specific requiments originated from clinical biomedicine, which can be realized by various synethic strategies such as covalent coupling, electrostatic absorption, layer-by-layer coating, etc. By optimizing the composition, structure, and morphology of MSNs-based biomaterials, their theranostic performance and biosafety can be further improved. For example, in addition to the delivery of traditional therapeutic agents, multifuncitonal mesoporous materials have found the applications in controlled drug releasing, targeted delivery, photodynamic therapy, synergistic therapy, antimetastasis of cancer cells, molecular imaging (e.g., MRI, fluorescent imaging, thermal imging, ultrasound imaging, computed tomography, photoacoustic imaging, radionuclide imaging, etc.), noninvasive therapy, etc. On this ground, this thesis aims to elaborately design, chemically synthesize, and extensively explore the biomedical applications of mesoporous silica biomaterials. We try our best to provide more efficient strategies to solve the critical issues for the early diagnosis and efficient therapy of serious diseases based on mesoporous silica-based biomaterials.

References

1. Smit B, Maesen TLM (2008) Molecular simulations of zeolites: adsorption, diffusion, and shape selectivity. Chem Rev 108(10):4125–4184
2. Cundy CS, Cox PA (2003) The hydrothermal synthesis of zeolites: history and development from the earliest days to the present time. Chem Rev 103(3):663–701
3. Kresge CT, Leonowicz ME, Roth WJ, Vartuli JC, Beck JS (1992) Ordered mesoporous molecular-sieves synthesized by a liquid-crystal template mechanism. Nature 359(6397):710–712
4. Corma A (1997) From microporous to mesoporous molecular sieve materials and their use in catalysis. Chem Rev 97(6):2373–2419
5. Davis ME (2002) Ordered porous materials for emerging applications. Nature 417(6891):813–821
6. Beck JS, Vartuli JC, Roth WJ, Leonowicz ME, Kresge CT, Schmitt KD, Chu CTW, Olson DH, Sheppard EW, McCullen SB, Higgins JB, Schlenker JL (1992) A new family of mesoporous molecular-sieves prepared with liquid-crystal templates. J Am Chem Soc 114(27):10834–10843
7. Zhao DY, Feng JL, Huo QS, Melosh N, Fredrickson GH, Chmelka BF, Stucky GD (1998) Triblock copolymer syntheses of mesoporous silica with periodic 50 to 300 angstrom pores. Science 279(5350):548–552
8. Kaneda M, Tsubakiyama T, Carlsson A, Sakamoto Y, Ohsuna T, Terasaki O, Joo SH, Ryoo R (2002) Structural study of mesoporous MCM-48 and carbon networks synthesized in the spaces of MCM-48 by electron crystallography. J Phys Chem B 106(6):1256–1266

9. Jun S, Joo SH, Ryoo R, Kruk M, Jaroniec M, Liu Z, Ohsuna T, Terasaki O (2000) Synthesis of new, nanoporous carbon with hexagonally ordered mesostructure. J Am Chem Soc 122(43):10712–10713

10. Wan Y, Zhao DY (2007) On the controllable soft-templating approach to mesoporous silicates. Chem Rev 107(7):2821–2860

11. Firouzi A, Kumar D, Bull LM, Besier T, Sieger P, Huo Q, Walker SA, Zasadzinski JA, Glinka C, Nicol J, Margolese D, Stucky GD, Chmelka BF (1995) Cooperative organization of inorganic-surfactant and biomimetic assemblies. Science 267(5201):1138–1143

12. Tian BZ, Liu XY, Tu B, Yu CZ, Fan J, Wang LM, Xie SH, Stucky GD, Zhao DY (2003) Self-adjusted synthesis of ordered stable mesoporous minerals by acid-base pairs. Nat Mater 2(3):159–163

13. Monnier A, Schuth F, Huo Q, Kumar D, Margolese D, Maxwell RS, Stucky GD, Krishnamurty M, Petroff P, Firouzi A, Janicke M, Chmelka BF (1993) Cooperative formation of inorganic-organic interfaces in the synthesis of silicate mesostructures. Science 261(5126):1299–1303

14. Israelachvili JN, Mitchell DJ, Ninham BW (1976) Theory of self-assembly of hydrocarbon amphiphiles into micelles and bilayers. J Chem Soc-Faraday Trans 72:1525–1568

15. Huo QS, Margolese DI, Stucky GD (1996) Surfactant control of phases in the synthesis of mesoporous silica-based materials. Chem Mater 8(5):1147–1160

16. Zhao DY, Huo QS, Feng JL, Kim JM, Han YJ, Stucky GD (1999) Novel mesoporous silicates with two-dimensional mesostructure direction using rigid bolaform surfactants. Chem Mater 11(10):2668–2672

17. Khushalani D, Kuperman A, Coombs N, Ozin GA (1996) Mixed surfactant assemblies in the synthesis of mesoporous silicas. Chem Mater 8(8):2188–2193

18. Kim JM, Sakamoto Y, Hwang YK, Kwon YU, Terasaki O, Park SE, Stucky GD (2002) Structural design of mesoporous silica by micelle-packing control using blends of amphiphilic block copolymers. J Phys Chem B 106(10):2552–2558

19. Yu CZ, Yu YH, Miao L, Zhao DY (2001) Highly ordered mesoporous silica structures templated by poly(butylene oxide) segment di- and tri-block copolymers. Microporous Mesoporous Mater 44:65–72

20. Huo QS, Margolese DI, Ciesla U, Feng PY, Gier TE, Sieger P, Leon R, Petroff PM, Schuth F, Stucky GD (1994) Generalized synthesis of periodic surfactant inorganic composite-materials. Nature 368(6469):317–321

21. Kim SS, Karkamkar A, Pinnavaia TJ, Kruk M, Jaroniec M (2001) Synthesis and characterization of ordered, very large pore MSU-H silicas assembled from water-soluble silicates. J Phys Chem B 105(32):7663–7670

22. El-Safty SA, Hanaoka T (2004) Microemulsion liquid crystal templates for highly ordered three-dimensional mesoporous silica monoliths with controllable mesopore structures. Chem Mater 16(3):384–400

23. El-Safty SA, Hanaoka T (2003) Monolithic nanostructured silicate family templated by lyotropic liquid-crystalline nonionic surfactant mesophases. Chem Mater 15(15):2892–2902

24. Zhang ZD, Tian BZ, Shen SD, Fan J, Tu B, Kong QY, Xiao FS, Qiu SL, Zhao DY (2002) Preparation of highly ordered well-defined single crystal cubic mesoporous silica templated by gemini surfactant. Chem Lett 6:584–585

25. Wang LM, Tian BZ, Fan J, Liu XY, Yang HF, Yu CZ, Tu B, Zhao DY (2004) Block copolymer templating syntheses of ordered large-pore stable mesoporous aluminophosphates and Fe-aluminophosphate based on an "acid-base pair" route. Microporous Mesoporous Mater 67(2–3):123–133

26. Ryoo R, Joo SH, Kim JM (1999) Energetically favored formation of MCM-48 from cationic-neutral surfactant mixtures. J Phys Chem B 103(35):7435–7440

27. Chen FX, Huang LM, Li QZ (1997) Synthesis of MCM-48 using mixed cationic-anionic surfactants as templates. Chem Mater 9(12):2685–2686

28. Attard GS, Glyde JC, Goltner CG (1995) Liquid-crystalline phases as templates for the synthesis of mesoporous silica. Nature 378(6555):366–368
29. Huo QS, Margolese DI, Ciesla U, Demuth DG, Feng PY, Gier TE, Sieger P, Firouzi A, Chmelka BF, Schuth F, Stucky GD (1994) Organization of organic-molecules with inorganic molecular-species into nanocomposite biphase arrays. Chem Mater 6(8):1176–1191
30. Zhao DY, Huo QS, Feng JL, Chmelka BF, Stucky GD (1998) Nonionic triblock and star diblock copolymer and oligomeric surfactant syntheses of highly ordered, hydrothermally stable, mesoporous silica structures. J Am Chem Soc 120(24):6024–6036
31. Inagaki S, Fukushima Y, Kuroda K (1993) Synthesis of highly ordered mesoporous materials from a layered polysilicate. J Chem Soc-Chem Commun 8:680–682
32. Gu JL, Shi JL, You GJ, Xiong LM, Qian SX, Hua ZL, Chen HR (2005) Incorporation of highly dispersed gold nanoparticles into the pore channels of mesoporous silica thin films and their ultrafast nonlinear optical response. Adv Mater 17(5):557–560
33. Liu XY, Tian BZ, Yu CZ, Gao F, Xie SH, Tu B, Che RC, Peng LM, Zhao DY (2002) Room-temperature synthesis in acidic media of large-pore three-dimensional bicontinuous mesoporous silica with Ia3d symmetry. Angew Chem-Int Edit 41(20):3876–3878
34. Goltner CG, Henke S, Weissenberger MC, Antonietti M (1998) Mesoporous silica from lyotropic liquid crystal polymer templates. Angew Chem-Int Edit 37(5):613–616
35. Huo QS, Leon R, Petroff PM, Stucky GD (1995) Mesostructure design with gemini surfactants - supercage formation in a 3-dimensional hexagonal array. Science 268(5215):1324–1327
36. Zhao D, Yang P, Melosh N, Feng J, Chmelka BF, Stucky GD (1998) Continuous mesoporous silica films with highly ordered large pore structures. Adv Mater 10(16):1380–1385
37. Bagshaw SA, Hayman AR (2000) Novel super-microporous silicate templating by omega-hydroxyalkylammonium halide bolaform surfactants. Chem Commun 7:533–534
38. El Haskouri J, Cabrera S, Caldes M, Guillem C, Latorre J, Beltran A, Beltran D, Marcos MD, Amoros P (2002) Surfactant-assisted synthesis of the SBA-8 mesoporous silica by using nonrigid commercial alkyltrimethyl ammonium surfactants. Chem Mater 14(6):2637–2643
39. Grosso D, Balkenende AR, Albouy PA, Ayral A, Amenitsch H, Babonneau F (2001) Two-dimensional hexagonal mesoporous silica thin films prepared from black copolymers: Detailed characterization amd formation mechanism. Chem Mater 13(5):1848–1856
40. Grosso D, Soler-Illia G, Babonneau F, Sanchez C, Albouy PA, Brunet-Bruneau A, Balkenende AR (2001) Highly organized mesoporous titania thin films showing mono-oriented 2D hexagonal channels. Adv Mater 13(14):1085–1090
41. Matos JR, Kruk M, Mercuri LP, Jaroniec M, Zhao L, Kamiyama T, Terasaki O, Pinnavaia TJ, Liu Y (2003) Ordered mesoporous silica with large cage-like pores: structural identification and pore connectivity design by controlling the synthesis temperature and time. J Am Chem Soc 125(3):821–829
42. Shen SD, Li YQ, Zhang ZD, Fan J, Tu B, Zhou WZ, Zhao DY (2002) A novel ordered cubic mesoporous silica templated with tri-head group quaternary ammonium surfactant. Chem Commun 19:2212–2213
43. Garcia-Bennett AE, Miyasaka K, Terasaki O, Che SN (2004) Structural solution of mesocaged material AMS-8. Chem Mater 16(19):3597–3605
44. Fan J, Yu CZ, Gao T, Lei J, Tian BZ, Wang LM, Luo Q, Tu B, Zhou WZ, Zhao DY (2003) Cubic mesoporous silica with large controllable entrance sizes and advanced adsorption properties. Angew Chem-Int Edit 42(27):3146–3150
45. Kleitz F, Liu DN, Anilkumar GM, Park IS, Solovyov LA, Shmakov AN, Ryoo R (2003) Large cage face-centered-cubic Fm3m mesoporous silica: Synthesis and structure. J Phys Chem B 107(51):14296–14300
46. Yanagisawa T, Shimizu T, Kuroda K, Kato C (1990) The preparation of alkyltrimethylammonium-kanemite complexes and their conversion to microporous materials. Bull Chem Soc Jpn 63(4):988–992

47. Inagaki S, Koiwai A, Suzuki N, Fukushima Y, Kuroda K (1996) Syntheses of highly ordered mesoporous materials, FSM-16, derived from kanemite. Bull Chem Soc Jpn 69(5):1449–1457

48. Tanev PT, Chibwe M, Pinnavaia TJ (1994) Titanium-containing mesoporous molecular-sieves for catalytic-oxidation of aromatic-compounds. Nature 368(6469):321–323

49. Tanev PT, Pinnavaia TJ (1995) A neutral templating route to mesoporous molecular-sieves. Science 267(5199):865–867

50. Ryoo R, Kim JM, Ko CH, Shin CH (1996) Disordered molecular sieve with branched mesoporous channel network. J Phys Chem 100(45):17718–17721

51. Jansen JC, Shan Z, Marchese L, Zhou W, von der Puil N, Maschmeyer T (2001) A new templating method for three-dimensional mesopore networks. Chem Commun 8:713–714

52. Che S, Liu Z, Ohsuna T, Sakamoto K, Terasaki O, Tatsumi T (2004) Synthesis and characterization of chiral mesoporous silica. Nature 429(6989):281–284

53. Kim SS, Zhang WZ, Pinnavaia TJ (1998) Ultrastable mesostructured silica vesicles. Science 282(5392):1302–1305

54. Yu CZ, Fan J, Tian BZ, Stucky GD, Zhao DY (2003) Synthesis of mesoporous silica from commercial poly(ethylene oxide)/poly(butylene oxide) copolymers: toward the rational design of ordered mesoporous materials. J Phys Chem B 107(48):13368–13375

55. Zhao WR, Lang MD, Li YS, Li L, Shi JL (2009) Fabrication of uniform hollow mesoporous silica spheres and ellipsoids of tunable size through a facile hard-templating route. J Mater Chem 19(18):2778–2783

56. Feng ZG, Li YS, Niu DC, Li L, Zhao WR, Chen HR, Gao JH, Ruan ML, Shi JL (2008) A facile route to hollow nanospheres of mesoporous silica with tunable size. Chem Commun 23:2629–2631

57. Li YS, Shi JL, Hua ZL, Chen HR, Ruan ML, Yan DS (2003) Hollow spheres of mesoporous aluminosilicate with a three-dimensional pore network and extraordinarily high hydrothermal stability. Nano Lett 3(5):609–612

58. Dong Y, Lin HM, Qu FY (2012) Synthesis of ferromagnetic ordered mesoporous carbons for bulky dye molecules adsorption. Chem Eng J 193:169–177

59. Guo LM, Zhang LX, Zhang JM, Zhou J, He QJ, Zeng SZ, Cui XZ, Shi JL (2009) Hollow mesoporous carbon spheres-an excellent bilirubin adsorbent. Chem Commun 40:6071–6073

60. Tao G, Zhang L, Hua Z, Chen Y, Guo L, Zhang J, Shu Z, Gao J, Chen H, Wu W, Liu Z, Shi J (2014) Highly efficient adsorbents based on hierarchically macro/mesoporous carbon monoliths with strong hydrophobicity. Carbon 66:547–559

61. Ryoo R, Joo SH, Kruk M, Jaroniec M (2001) Ordered mesoporous carbons. Adv Mater 13(9):677–681

62. Chen Y, Chen HR, Guo LM, He QJ, Chen F, Zhou J, Feng JW, Shi JL (2010) Hollow/Rattle-type mesoporous nanostructures by a structural difference-based selective etching strategy. ACS Nano 4(1):529–539

63. Zhao WR, Chen HR, Li YS, Li L, Lang MD, Shi JL (2008) Uniform Rattle-type hollow magnetic mesoporous spheres as drug delivery carriers and their sustained-release property. Adv Funct Mater 18(18):2780–2788

64. Vallet-Regi M, Ramila A, del Real RP, Perez-Pariente J (2001) A new property of MCM-41: drug delivery system. Chem Mater 13(2):308–311

65. Vallet-Regi M, Balas F, Arcos D (2007) Mesoporous materials for drug delivery. Angew Chem-Int Edit 46(40):7548–7558

66. Horcajada P, Ramila A, Perez-Pariente J, Vallet-Regi M (2004) Influence of pore size of MCM-41 matrices on drug delivery rate. Microporous Mesoporous Mater 68(1–3):105–109

67. Zhu YF, Shi JL, Chen HR, Shen WH, Dong XP (2005) A facile method to synthesize novel hollow mesoporous silica spheres and advanced storage property. Microporous Mesoporous Mater 84(1–3):218–222

68. Zhu YF, Shi JL, Shen WH, Dong XP, Feng JW, Ruan ML, Li YS (2005) Stimuli-responsive controlled drug release from a hollow mesoporous silica sphere/polyelectrolyte multilayer core-shell structure. Angew Chem-Int Edit 44(32):5083–5087

69. Singh N, Karambelkar A, Gu L, Lin K, Miller JS, Chen CS, Sailor MJ, Bhatia SN (2011) Bioresponsive mesoporous silica nanoparticles for triggered drug release. J Am Chem Soc 133(49):19582–19585

70. Vivero-Escoto JL, Slowing II, Trewyn BG, Lin VSY (2010) Mesoporous silica nanoparticles for intracellular controlled drug delivery. Small 6(18):1952–1967

71. Du J-Z, Sun T-M, Song W-J, Wu J, Wang J (2010) A Tumor-Acidity-Activated Charge-Conversional Nanogel as an Intelligent Vehicle for Promoted Tumoral-Cell Uptake and Drug Delivery. Angew Chem-Int Edit 49(21):3621–3626

72. Lee ES, Gao ZG, Bae YH (2008) Recent progress in tumor pH targeting nanotechnology. J Control Release 132(3):164–170

73. Mal NK, Fujiwara M, Tanaka Y (2003) Photocontrolled reversible release of guest molecules from coumarin-modified mesoporous silica. Nature 421(6921):350–353

74. Vivero-Escoto JL, Slowing II, Wu CW, Lin VSY (29009) Photoinduced intracellular controlled release drug delivery in human cells by gold-capped mesoporous silica nanosphere. J Am Chem Soc 131(10):3462

75. Lai JP, Mu X, Xu YY, Wu XL, Wu CL, Li C, Chen JB, Zhao YB (2010) Light-responsive nanogated ensemble based on polymer grafted mesoporous silica hybrid nanoparticles. Chem Commun 46(39):7370–7372

76. Ferris DP, Zhao YL, Khashab NM, Khatib HA, Stoddart JF, Zink JI (2009) Light-operated mechanized nanoparticles. J Am Chem Soc 131(5):1686

77. Knezevic NZ, Trewyn BG, Lin VSY (2011) Functionalized mesoporous silica nanoparticle-based visible light responsive controlled release delivery system. Chem Commun 47(10):2817–2819

78. Lin QN, Huang Q, Li CY, Bao CY, Liu ZZ, Li FY, Zhu LY (2010) Anticancer drug release from a mesoporous silica based nanophotocage regulated by either a one- or two-photon process. J Am Chem Soc 132(31):10645–10647

79. Aznar E, Marcos MD, Martinez-Manez R, Sancenon F, Soto J, Amoros P, Guillem C (2009) pH- and photo-switched release of guest molecules from mesoporous silica supports. J Am Chem Soc 131(19):6833–6843

80. Yang Q, Wang SH, Fan PW, Wang LF, Di Y, Lin KF, Xiao FS (2005) pH-responsive carrier system based on carboxylic acid modified mesoporous silica and polyelectrolyte for drug delivery. Chem Mater 17(24):5999–6003

81. Park C, Oh K, Lee SC, Kim C (2007) Controlled release of guest molecules from mesoporous silica particles based on a pH-responsive polypseudorotaxane motif. Angew Chem-Int Edit 46(9):1455–1457

82. Sun JT, Hong CY, Pan CY (2010) Fabrication of PDEAEMA-coated mesoporous silica nanoparticles and pH-responsive controlled release. J Phys Chem C 114(29):12481–12486

83. Lee CH, Cheng SH, Huang IP, Souris JS, Yang CS, Mou CY, Lo LW (2010) Intracellular pH-responsive mesoporous silica nanoparticles for the controlled release of anticancer chemotherapeutics. Angew Chem-Int Edit 49(44):8214–8219

84. Chen CE, Pu F, Huang ZZ, Liu Z, Ren JS, Qu XG (2011) Stimuli-responsive controlled-release system using quadruplex DNA-capped silica nanocontainers. Nucleic Acids Res 39(4):1638–1644

85. Gao Q, Xu Y, Wu D, Sun YH, Li XA (2009) pH-responsive drug release from polymer-coated mesoporous silica spheres. J Phys Chem C 113(29):12753–12758

86. Hong C-Y, Li X, Pan C-Y (2009) Fabrication of smart nanocontainers with a mesoporous core and a pH-responsive shell for controlled uptake and release. J Mater Chem 19(29):5155–5160

87. Giri S, Trewyn BG, Stellmaker MP, Lin VSY (2005) Stimuli-responsive controlled-release delivery system based on mesoporous silica nanorods capped with magnetic nanoparticles. Angew Chem-Int Edit 44(32):5038–5044

88. Lai CY, Trewyn BG, Jeftinija DM, Jeftinija K, Xu S, Jeftinija S, Lin VSY (2003) A mesoporous silica nanosphere-based carrier system with chemically removable CdS nanoparticle caps for stimuli-responsive controlled release of neurotransmitters and drug molecules. J Am Chem Soc 125(15):4451–4459

89. Liu R, Zhao X, Wu T, Feng PY (2008) Tunable redox-responsive hybrid nanogated ensembles. J Am Chem Soc 130(44):14418–14419

90. Bernardos A, Aznar E, Marcos MD, Martinez-Manez R, Sancenon F, Soto J, Barat JM, Amoros P (2009) Enzyme-responsive controlled release using mesoporous silica supports capped with lactose. Angew Chem-Int Edit 48(32):5884–5887

91. Bernardos A, Mondragon L, Aznar E, Marcos MD, Martinez-Manez R, Sancenon F, Soto J, Barat JM, Perez-Paya E, Guillem C, Amoros P (2010) Enzyme-responsive intracellular controlled release using nanometric silica mesoporous supports capped with "Saccharides". ACS Nano 4(11):6353–6368

92. Coll C, Mondragon L, Martinez-Manez R, Sancenon F, Marcos MD, Soto J, Amoros P, Perez-Paya E (2011) Enzyme-mediated controlled release systems by anchoring peptide sequences on mesoporous silica supports. Angew Chem-Int Edit 50(9):2138–2140

93. Patel K, Angelos S, Dichtel WR, Coskun A, Yang YW, Zink JI, Stoddart JF (2008) Enzyme-responsive snap-top covered silica nanocontainers. J Am Chem Soc 130(8):2382–2383

94. Park C, Kim H, Kim S, Kim C (2009) Enzyme responsive nanocontainers with cyclodextrin gatekeepers and synergistic effects in release of guests. J Am Chem Soc 131(46):16614–16615

95. Schlossbauer A, Kecht J, Bein T (2009) Biotin-avidin as a protease-responsive cap system for controlled guest release from colloidal mesoporous silica. Angew Chem-Int Edit 48(17):3092–3095

96. You YZ, Kalebaila KK, Brock SL, Oupicky D (2008) Temperature-controlled uptake and release in PNIPAM-modified porous silica nanoparticles. Chem Mater 20(10):3354–3359

97. Liu CY, Guo J, Yang WL, Hu JH, Wang CC, Fu SK (2009) Magnetic mesoporous silica microspheres with thermo-sensitive polymer shell for controlled drug release. J Mater Chem 19(27):4764–4770

98. Zhu YF, Kaskel S, Ikoma T, Hanagata N (2009) Magnetic SBA-15/poly(N-isopropylacrylamide) composite: preparation, characterization and temperature-responsive drug release property. Microporous Mesoporous Mater 123(1–3):107–112

99. Climent E, Bernardos A, Martinez-Manez R, Maquieira A, Marcos MD, Pastor-Navarro N, Puchades R, Sancenon F, Soto J, Amoros P (2009) Controlled delivery systems using antibody-capped mesoporous nanocontainers. J Am Chem Soc 131(39):14075–14080

100. Zhao YN, Trewyn BG, Slowing II, Lin VSY (2009) Mesoporous silica nanoparticle-based double drug delivery system for glucose-responsive controlled release of insulin and cyclic AMP. J Am Chem Soc 131(24):8398–8400

101. Kim HJ, Matsuda H, Zhou HS, Honma I (2006) Ultrasound-triggered smart drug release from a poly(dimethylsiloxane)-mesoporous silica composite. Adv Mater 18(23):3083–3088

102. Ren CL, Li JH, Chen XG, Hu ZD, Xue DS (2007) Preparation and properties of a new multifunctional material composed of superparamagnetic core and rhodamine B doped silica shell. Nanotechnology 18(34):6

103. Cheng S-H, Lee C-H, Yang C-S, Tseng F-G, Mou C-Y, Lo L-W (2009) Mesoporous silica nanoparticles functionalized with an oxygen-sensing probe for cell photodynamic therapy: potential cancer theranostics. J Mater Chem 19(9):1252–1257

104. Yang Y, Song W, Wang A, Zhu P, Fei J, Li J (2010) Lipid coated mesoporous silica nanoparticles as photosensitive drug carriers. Phys Chem Chem Phys 12(17):4418–4422

105. Lee SM, O'Halloran TV, Nguyen ST (2010) Polymer-caged nanobins for synergistic cisplatin-doxorubicin combination chemotherapy. J Am Chem Soc 132(48):17130–17138

106. Chen AM, Zhang M, Wei DG, Stueber D, Taratula O, Minko T, He HX (2009) Co-delivery of Doxorubicin and Bcl-2 siRNA by mesoporous silica nanoparticles enhances the efficacy of chemotherapy in multidrug-resistant cancer cells. Small 5(23):2673–2677

107. Meng HA, Liong M, Xia TA, Li ZX, Ji ZX, Zink JI, Nel AE (2010) Engineered design of mesoporous silica nanoparticles to deliver doxorubicin and P-glycoprotein siRNA to overcome drug resistance in a cancer cell line. ACS Nano 4(8):4539–4550
108. He QJ, Gao Y, Zhang LX, Zhang ZW, Gao F, Ji XF, Li YP, Shi JL (2011) A pH-responsive mesoporous silica nanoparticles-based multi-drug delivery system for overcoming multi-drug resistance. Biomaterials 32(30):7711–7720
109. Rosenholm JM, Meinander A, Peuhu E, Niemi R, Eriksson JE, Sahlgren C, Linden M (2009) Targeting of porous hybrid silica nanoparticles to cancer cells. ACS Nano 3(1):197–206
110. Pan LM, He QJ, Liu JN, Chen Y, Ma M, Zhang LL, Shi JL (2012) Nuclear-targeted drug delivery of TAT peptide-conjugated monodisperse mesoporous silica nanoparticles. J Am Chem Soc 134(13):5722–5725
111. Tsai CP, Chen CY, Hung Y, Chang FH, Mou CY (2009) Monoclonal antibody-functionalized mesoporous silica nanoparticles (MSN) for selective targeting breast cancer cells. J Mater Chem 19(32):5737–5743
112. Zhu CL, Song XY, Zhou WH, Yang HH, Wen YH, Wang XR (2009) An efficient cell-targeting and intracellular controlled-release drug delivery system based on MSN-PEM-aptamer conjugates. J Mater Chem 19(41):7765–7770
113. Ma M, Chen HR, Chen Y, Zhang K, Wang X, Cui XZ, Shi JL (2012) Hyaluronic acid-conjugated mesoporous silica nanoparticles: excellent colloidal dispersity in physiological fluids and targeting efficacy. J Mater Chem 22(12):5615–5621
114. Liong M, Lu J, Kovochich M, Xia T, Ruehm SG, Nel AE, Tamanoi F, Zink JI (2008) Multifunctional inorganic nanoparticles for imaging, targeting, and drug delivery. ACS Nano 2(5):889–896
115. Kim J, Kim HS, Lee N, Kim T, Kim H, Yu T, Song IC, Moon WK, Hyeon T (2008) Multifunctional uniform nanoparticles composed of a magnetite nanocrystal core and a mesoporous silica shell for magnetic resonance and fluorescence imaging and for drug delivery. Angew Chem-Int Edit 47(44):8438–8441
116. Knezevic NZ, Ruiz-Hernandez E, Hennink WE, Vallet-Regi M (2013) Magnetic mesoporous silica-based core/shell nanoparticles for biomedical applications. RSC Adv 3(25):9584–9593
117. Zhao WR, Gu JL, Zhang LX, Chen HR, Shi JL (2005) Fabrication of uniform magnetic nanocomposite spheres with a magnetic core/mesoporous silica shell structure. J Am Chem Soc 127(25):8916–8917
118. Deng Y, Qi D, Deng C, Zhang X, Zhao D (2008) Superparamagnetic high-magnetization microspheres with an $Fe_3O_4@SiO_2$ core and perpendicularly aligned mesoporous SiO_2 shell for removal of microcystins. J Am Chem Soc 130(1):28–29
119. Kim J, Lee JE, Lee J, Yu JH, Kim BC, An K, Hwang Y, Shin CH, Park JG, Hyeon T (2006) Magnetic fluorescent delivery vehicle using uniform mesoporous silica spheres embedded with monodisperse magnetic and semiconductor nanocrystals. J Am Chem Soc 128(3):688–689
120. Lee JE, Lee N, Kim H, Kim J, Choi SH, Kim JH, Kim T, Song IC, Park SP, Moon WK, Hyeon T (2010) Uniform mesoporous dye-doped silica nanoparticles decorated with multiple magnetite nanocrystals for simultaneous enhanced magnetic resonance imaging, fluorescence imaging, and drug delivery. J Am Chem Soc 132(2):552–557
121. Gan Q, Lu X, Yuan Y, Qian J, Zhou H, Lu X, Shi J, Liu C (2011) A magnetic, reversible pH-responsive nanogated ensemble based on Fe_3O_4 nanoparticles-capped mesoporous silica. Biomaterials 32(7):1932–1942
122. Viswanathan S, Kovacs Z, Green KN, Ratnakar SJ, Sherry AD (2010) Alternatives to Gadolinium-based metal chelates for magnetic resonance imaging. Chem Rev 110(5):2960–3018
123. Terreno E, Castelli DD, Viale A, Aime S (2010) Challenges for molecular magnetic resonance imaging. Chem Rev 110(5):3019–3042

124. Taylor KML, Kim JS, Rieter WJ, An H, Lin WL, Lin WB (2008) Mesoporous silica nano-spheres as highly efficient MRI contrast agents. J Am Chem Soc 130(7):2154–2155
125. Hsiao JK, Tsai CP, Chung TH, Hung Y, Yao M, Liu HM, Mou CY, Yang CS, Chen YC, Huang DM (2008) Mesoporous silica nanoparticles as a delivery system of gadolinium for effective human stem cell tracking. Small 4(9):1445–1452
126. Penfield JG, Reilly RF (2007) What nephrologists need to know about gadolinium. Nat Clin Pract Nephrol 3(12):654–668
127. Tromsdorf UI, Bruns OT, Salmen SC, Beisiegel U, Weller H (2009) A highly effective, non-toxic T-1 MR contrast agent based on ultrasmall pegylated iron oxide nanoparticles. Nano Lett 9(12):4434–4440
128. Perez-Rodriguez J, Lai S, Ehst BD, Fine DM, Bluemke DA (2009) Nephrogenic systemic fibrosis: incidence, associations, and effect of risk factor assessment-report of 33 cases. Radiology 250(2):371–377
129. Na HB, Lee JH, An KJ, Park YI, Park M, Lee IS, Nam DH, Kim ST, Kim SH, Kim SW, Lim KH, Kim KS, Kim SO, Hyeon T (2007) Development of a T-1 contrast agent for magnetic resonance imaging using MnO nanoparticles. Angew Chem-Int Edit 46(28):5397–5401
130. Peng Y-K, Lai C-W, Liu C-L, Chen H-C, Hsiao Y-H, Liu W-L, Tang K-C, Chi Y, Hsiao J-K, Lim K-E, Liao H-E, Shyue J-J, Chou P-T (2011) A new and facile method to pre-pare uniform hollow MnO/functionalized mSiO(2) core/shell nanocomposites. ACS Nano 5(5):4177–4187
131. Schladt TD, Shukoor MI, Schneider K, Tahir MN, Natalio F, Ament I, Becker J, Jochum FD, Weber S, Kohler O, Theato P, Schreiber LM, Sonnichsen C, Schroder HC, Muller WEG, Tremel W (2010) Au@MnO Nanoflowers: hybrid nanocomposites for selective dual functionalization and imaging. Angew Chem-Int Edit 49(23):3976–3980
132. Kim T, Momin E, Choi J, Yuan K, Zaidi H, Kim J, Park M, Lee N, McMahon MT, Quinones-Hinojosa A, Bulte JWM, Hyeon T, Gilad AA (2011) Mesoporous silica-coated hollow manganese oxide nanoparticles as positive T-1 contrast agents for labeling and MRI tracking of adipose-derived mesenchymal stem cells. J Am Chem Soc 133(9):2955–2961
133. Liu JA, Bu WB, Zhang SJ, Chen F, Xing HY, Pan LM, Zhou LP, Peng WJ, Shi JL (2012) Controlled synthesis of uniform and monodisperse upconversion core/mesoporous silica shell nanocomposites for bimodal imaging. Chem-Eur J 18(8):2335–2341
134. He QJ, Shi JL, Cui XZ, Wei CY, Zhang LX, Wu W, Bu WB, Chen HR, Wu HX (2011) Synthesis of oxygen-deficient luminescent mesoporous silica nanoparticles for synchronous drug delivery and imaging. Chem Commun 47(28):7947–7949
135. He QJ, Ma M, Wei CY, Shi JL (2012) Mesoporous carbon@silicon-silica nanotheranos-tics for synchronous delivery of insoluble drugs and luminescence imaging. Biomaterials 33(17):4392–4402
136. Erogbogbo F, Yong K-T, Roy I, Xu G, Prasad PN, Swihart MT (2008) Biocompatible lumi-nescent silicon quantum dots for imaging of cancer cells. ACS Nano 2(5):873–878
137. Gupta A, Swihart MT, Wiggers H (2009) Luminescent colloidal dispersion of silicon quan-tum dots from microwave plasma synthesis: exploring the photoluminescence behavior across the visible spectrum. Adv Funct Mater 19(5):696–703
138. Bruchez M, Moronne M, Gin P, Weiss S, Alivisatos AP (1998) Semiconductor nanocrystals as fluorescent biological labels. Science 281(5385):2013–2016
139. Michalet X, Pinaud FF, Bentolila LA, Tsay JM, Doose S, Li JJ, Sundaresan G, Wu AM, Gambhir SS, Weiss S (2005) Quantum dots for live cells, in vivo imaging, and diagnostics. Science 307(5709):538–544
140. Sun Y, Yu M, Liang S, Zhang Y, Li C, Mou T, Yang W, Zhang X, Li B, Huang C, Li F (2011) Fluorine-18 labeled rare-earth nanoparticles for positron emission tomography (PET) imag-ing of sentinel lymph node. Biomaterials 32(11):2999–3007
141. Xiong LQ, Yang TS, Yang Y, Xu CJ, Li FY (2010) Long-term in vivo biodistribution imag-ing and toxicity of polyacrylic acid-coated upconversion nanophosphors. Biomaterials 31(27):7078–7085

142. Gai S, Yang P, Li C, Wang W, Dai Y, Niu N, Lin J (2010) Synthesis of magnetic, up-conversion luminescent, and mesoporous core-shell-structured nanocomposites as drug carriers. Adv Funct Mater 20(7):1166–1172
143. Lee CH, Cheng SH, Wang YJ, Chen YC, Chen NT, Souris J, Chen CT, Mou CY, Yang CS, Lo LW (2009) Near-infrared mesoporous silica nanoparticles for optical imaging: characterization and in vivo biodistribution. Adv Funct Mater 19(2):215–222
144. Pan J, Wan D, Gong JL (2011) PEGylated liposome coated QDs/mesoporous silica core-shell nanoparticles for molecular imaging. Chem Commun 47(12):3442–3444
145. Qian HS, Guo HC, Ho PCL, Mahendran R, Zhang Y (2009) Mesoporous-silica-coated up-conversion fluorescent nanoparticles for photodynamic therapy. Small 5(20):2285–2290
146. Feng J, Song S-Y, Deng R-P, Fan W-Q, Zhang H-J (2010) Novel multifunctional nano-composites: magnetic mesoporous silica nanospheres covalently bonded with near-infrared luminescent lanthanide complexes. Langmuir 26(5):3596–3600
147. Chen Y, Chen HR, Zhang SJ, Chen F, Zhang LX, Zhang JM, Zhu M, Wu HX, Guo LM, Feng JW, Shi JL (2011) Multifunctional mesoporous nanoellipsoids for biological bimodal imaging and magnetically targeted delivery of anticancer drugs. Adv Funct Mater 21(2):270–278
148. Ma M, Chen HR, Chen Y, Wang X, Chen F, Cui XZ, Shi JL (2012) Au capped magnetic core/mesoporous silica shell nanoparticles for combined photothermo-/chemo-therapy and multimodal imaging. Biomaterials 33(3):989–998

Chapter 2
Synthesis of Hollow Mesoporous Silica Nanoparticles by Silica-Etching Chemistry for Biomedical Applications

2.1 Introduction

With the fast development of mesoporous materials for biomedical applications, many requirements on the morphology and structure of materials have been proposed [1−3]. Scientists need to design and fabricate mesoporous nanomaterials with unique functionalities based on the principles of chemical synthesis. Numerous studies have demonstrated that the performance of mesoporous silica-based material systems is strongly related to the composition, morphology, and structure of fabricated materials [4−7]. Therefore, mesoporous silica with diverse morphologies have been designed and synthesized, such as spherical, rod, fiber, tube, sheet, polyhedral shape, etc. [8]. The regulation of the morphologies of mesoporous silica is important in nanomedicine and nanobiotechnology because mesoporous silica nanoparticles (MSNs) with different morphologies show significantly different biological behaviors [9−11]. In addition, the particle sizes of MSNs strongly influence their in vivo bio-distributions and excretions [12, 13].

Among MSNs with abundant morphologies and nanostructures, hollow mesoporous silica nanoparticles (designated as HMSNs) have attracted tremendous attentions due to their unique hollow and mesoporous nanostructure [14−17]. The large hollow interiors of HMSNs leave more room for the loading of guest molecules compared to traditional MSNs. Thus, HMSNs show the high drug-loading capacity. The well-defined mesopores within the shell provide the diffusion path for guest molecules. In addition, the abundant surface chemistry of HMSNs make the surface engineering/modification possible such as PEGylation or targeting modification. On this ground, it is of high significance to design and fabricate HMSNs based on the principle of organic–inorganic nanosynthetic chemistry. Prof. Shi's group is one of the earliest research teams to prepare MSNs with large hollow interior and ordered mesopores [18, 19]. Their preliminary applications in biomedicine were also conducted. It was found that the large

© Springer-Verlag Berlin Heidelberg 2016
Y. Chen, *Design, Synthesis, Multifunctionalization and Biomedical Applications of Multifunctional Mesoporous Silica-Based Drug Delivery Nanosystems*,
Springer Theses, DOI 10.1007/978-3-662-48622-1_2

hollow interior of HMSNs could significantly enhance the drug-loading capability. For instance, the drug-loading amount of HMSNs toward ibuprofen (IBU) could reach as high as 744.5 mg/g, while traditional MCM-41-type MSNs without the hollow structure only encapsulated 358.6 mg IBU per gram MSNs [19].

However, there are still no simple, efficient, economic, and environment-friendly synthetic strategies to fabricate HMSNs with high dispersity, tunable particle size, and controllable mesopore size. In addition, the research on the biomedical applications of HMSNs is much less than that of MSNs. The most representative method to prepare HMSNs is so-called "templating method" [20]. Typically, such a templating method initially employs various soft/hard templates as the substrate, followed by coating a shell with desirable composition/structure onto the surface of the templates. After removing the templates, the hollow spheres can be obtained. Generally, the chemical composition between the core and shell is different, causing the different physiochemical properties. Based on these different physiochemical properties, the core template can be completely removed while the shell keeps intact by various physical or chemical approaches. In this chapter, we successfully developed a new templating method to prepare HMSNs, but the templating principle is not the traditional composition difference between the core and shell. We found that the structural differences between the core and shell could also be employed for the fabrication of HMSNs, though the chemical composition between the core and shell was the same with each other. We defined this method as "structural difference-based selective etching" (SDSE) strategy. Based on SDSE strategy, we successfully constructed HMSNs with desirable structure, composition and, physicochemical property. The formation mechanism and principle of HMSNs based on SDSE strategy were systematically investigated. We further studied the biological behaviors of HMSNs, including cytotoxicity and in vitro hemocompatibility. In addition, the specific function of HMSNs for in vitro anticancer drug delivery was revealed.

2.2 Experimental Section

2.2.1 Synthesis of HMSNs Based on SDSE Strategy

The fabrication of HMSNs includes three steps, i.e., fabrication of solid SiO_2 as the hard template, coating the SiO_2 template by mesoporous silica, and the final removal of SiO_2 template by chemical etching. Typically, ethanol (142.8 mL), H_2O (20 mL), and ammonia solution (3.14 mL) were premixed, followed by adding tetraethyl orthosilicate (TEOS, 6 mL) under magnetic stirring at 30 °C. After further 1 h reaction, the mixture of TEOS and octadecyltrimethoxysilane ($C_{18}TMS$) was added for another 6 h reaction. The product was collected by centrifugation and divided into six parts. Each part was etched in Na_2CO_3 solution (0.6 M, 50 mL) for 0.5 h at 80 °C. The etched sample was collected by centrifugation and washed several times by water and ethanol. After drying under vacuum at room temperature, the sample was calcined at 550 °C for 6 h to remove the organic part.

2.2.2 Synthesis of HMSNs by Chemical Etching in Ammonia Solution

The fabrication of HMSNs in ammonia solution was similar to the etching procedure in Na_2CO_3 solution. When $sSiO_2@mSiO_2$ was ready, they were dispersed into diluted ammonia solution (70 mL, 0.12 M or 0.24 M). They were further transferred into Teflon-lined stainless steel autoclave, which was treated at 150 °C for 24 h. When the autoclave was cooled down to room temperature, the product was collected by centrifugation and dried under vacuum. The sample was finally calcined at 550 °C for 6 h

2.2.3 Study of the Formation Mechanism of HMSNs

A: Synthesis of Stöber method-based SiO_2 nanoparticles

TEOS (6 mL) was directly added into the mixture of ethanol (142.8 mL), H_2O (20 mL), and ammonia solution (3.14 m) at 30 °C under magnetic stirring. After further 2 h reaction, the product was collected by centrifugation, washed by ethanol three times, and finally dried under vacuum at room temperature.

B: Synthesis of MSNs templated by $C_{18}TMS$

Ethanol (142.8 m), H_2O (20 mL), and ammonium solution (3.14 mL) were premixed and stirred at 30 °C, followed by adding the mixture of TEOS (5 mL) and $C_{18}TMS$ (2 mL). After further reaction at 30 °C for 1 h, the sample was collected by centrifugation, washed by ethanol three times, and dried under vacuum at room temperature.

2.2.4 Synthesis of Multifunctional Rattle-Type HMSNs Based on SDSE Strategy

A. $Au@mSiO_2$

Au nanoparticles were initially synthesized by heating $HAuCl_4 \cdot 3H_2O$ solution (18.0 mg in 30 mL water) at 100 °C under vigorous stirring, followed by adding sodium citrate solution as the reducing agent for another 30 min reaction. The surface of as-synthesized Au nanoparticles was coated by PVP10 (Polyvinylpyrrolidone, 12.8 g/L, and 0.235 mL) to facilitate the subsequent coating process. The PVP-modified Au nanoparticles were redispersed into water

(3.0 mL) by mild ultrasound treatment. Then, Au solution (1.0 mL) was added into a mixture solution with ammonia solution (0.62 mL), ethanol (13.6 mL), and H_2O (3.3 mL), followed by the addition of TEOS (0.86 mL) in ethanol (9.2 mL) under vigorous magnetic stirring. After further 1 h reaction, TEOS (0.714 mL) and $C_{18}TMS$ (0.286) mixture were directly added into above solution under vigorous stirring, which further lasted for another 1 h. The product was collected by centrifugation and washed by ethanol and water for several times. After drying at 100 °C, the sample was calcined at 500 °C for 6 h.

B. Fe_2O_3@$mSiO_2$ and Fe_3O_4@$mSiO_2$

Ellipsoidal Fe_2O_3 nanoparticles were initially synthesized by a hydrothermal method. Typically, $Fe(ClO_4)_3 \cdot 6H_2O$ (11.6 g), urea (1.5 g), and NaH_2PO_4 (0.16 g) were dissolved into deionized water (250 mL) to form a homogeneous solution, which was further transferred into an oven and incubated at 100 °C for 24 h. The product was collected by centrifugation and dried for further use. For the coating process, the as-synthesized Fe_3O_4 (30 mg) was dispersed into the solution containing ethanol (71.4 mL), H_2O (10 mL), and ammonia solution (3.14 mL), followed by adding TEOS (0.53 mL TEOS in 4.7 mL ethanol) at the speed of 4 mL/h. Then, the mixture of TEOS (0.3 mL) and $C_{18}TMS$ (0.2 mL) were added into the reaction system dropwise. The product was collected by centrifugation and washed by ethanol and water several times. The as-synthesized Fe_2O_3@SiO_2@$mSiO_2$ was treated in ammonia solution (0.12 M) at 150 °C for 24 h. After centrifugation and washing steps, the sample was dried and calcined at 550 °C for 6 h. The inner core of Fe_3O_4@$mSiO_2$ was reduced into Fe_3O_4 nanocrystals by the thermal treatment in mixed H_2 (5 % in volume) and Ar (95 % in volume) gases at 410 °C for 5 h.

2.2.5 Hemolytic Effect Evaluation

The red blood cells (RBCs) were kindly provided by Shanghai Blood Center, which was diluted to 1/10 of their initial volume by PBS for assessment. Typically, the RBCs suspension (0.3 mL) was co-incubated with (a) 1.2 mL PBS as the negative control, (b) 1.2 mL deionized water as the positive control, and (c) 1.2 mL HMSNs PBS suspensions at different concentrations (from 25 to 200 μg/mL). After the co-incubation for 2 h, the cells were centrifuged, and the supernatants were collected for UV-vis characterizations at $\lambda = 541$ nm to determine the hemolytic percentage.

2.2.6 In Vitro DOX-Loading into HMSNs

HMSNs (50 mg) were dispersed into DOX PBS solution (6 mL, 0.5 mg/mL) by mild ultrasound treatment. After stirring for 24 h in the dark, the DOX-loaded HMSNs were collected by centrifugation, which was dried under vacuum at room temperature. To determine the DOX-loading amount, the supernatant was collected for UV-vis test at $\lambda = 480$ nm.

2.2.7 MTT Evaluation of the Cytotoxicity of HMSNs and DOX-HMSNs

In vitro cytotoxicity of HMSNs and DOX-HMSNs was evaluated by a typical MTT method. MCF-7 breast cancer cells were initially seeded into a 96-well plate at the density of 2000 cells/well, which were cultured in 5 % CO_2 at 37 °C for 24 h. Free DOX and DOX-loaded HMSNs dispersed into the cell-culturing medium were used to substitute the initial solution. The adopted DOX concentrations are 0.02, 0.2, 2, and 10 μM. After the co-incubation for 24 h, the cell-culturing medium was replaced by MTT solution (0.8 mg/mL, 100 μL/well), followed by another co-incubation for 4 h. Finally, the MTT solution was replaced by dimethyl sulfoxide (DMSO, 100 μL/well), and the absorbance was recorded by a microplate reader (Bio-TekELx800) at the wavelength of 490 nm. The cytotoxicities of MCF-7 cells were expressed as the percentage of cell viability compared to the cells without the treatment.

2.3 Results and Discussion

2.3.1 Synthesis and Characterization of HMSNs

Based on mature Stöber method, silica nanoparticles (designated as SNs) with high dispersity could be easily obtained [21]. The syntheses of mesoporous silica nanoparticles (MSNs) are typically based on sol-gel chemistry, which employs surfactants or block copolymers as the structural directing agents to generate the mesopores. We anticipated that some structural differences would be present between these two silica-based nanoparticles, though they have almost the same chemical composition.

TEM image shows that the as-synthesized SNs (Fig. 2.1a) exhibit smooth surface and spherical morphology, while the prepared MSNs (Fig. 2.1b) have the rough surface and mesopores. In FTIR spectra (Fig. 2.1c), MSNs show that a red shift from 1101 to 1086 cm^{-1} occurs in the transverse-optical mode of Si–O–Si asymmetric stretching vibration band compared to SNs. Such a red shift indicates that MSNs have a more open structure and higher condensation degree of silica species. In ^{29}Si MAS NMR spectra (Fig. 2.1d), there are three distinctive signals at –92, –101 and –111 ppm, which can be indexed to $Q^2[(SiO)_2Si(OH)_2]$, $Q^3[(SiO)_3SiOH]$, and $Q^4[(SiO)_4Si]$ species, respectively. The calculated $Q^4/(Q^2 + Q^3)$ ratio of MSNs is much higher than that of SNs, indicating that MSNs have enhanced condensation degree compared to SNs [14].

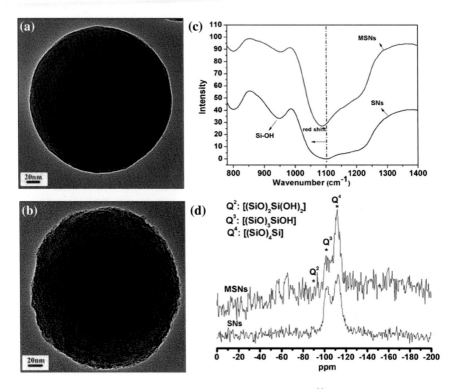

Fig. 2.1 TEM images of SNs (**a**) and MSNs (**b**); FTIR (**c**) and ^{29}Si MAS NMR (**d**) spectra of SNs and MSNs. Reproduced with permission from Ref. [28]. © 2010, American Chemical Society

To validate this idea, we used the layer-by-layer coating procedure to coat a mesoporous silica layer onto the surface of solid silica nanoparticles (sSiO$_2$@mSiO$_2$) · N$_2$CO$_3$ and ammonia solution were chosen as two alkaline etchants to etch sSiO$_2$@mSiO$_2$ nanoparticles. The evolution of the morphology and structure of hollow nanoparticles during the etching process can be observed by TEM images. As shown in Fig. 2.2a, the as-synthesized sSiO$_2$@mSiO$_2$ nanoparticles display the high dispersity and apparent core/shell structure. After the etching of sSiO$_2$@mSiO$_2$ in Na$_2$CO$_3$ solution (0.6 M) at 80 °C for 0.5 h, the core of sSiO$_2$@mSiO$_2$ could be completely etched away while the mesoporous silica shell are kept intact (Fig. 2.2b), by which highly dispersed HMSNs could be fabricated. After the treatment of sSiO$_2$@mSiO$_2$ within ammonia solution (0.12 M) at 150 °C for 24 h, the typical rattle-type HMSNs could be synthesized (Figs. 2.2c and 2.3). Further increase of the concentration of ammonia solution (from 0.12 to 0.24 M) completely removed the inner SiO$_2$ core to produce HMSNs, as shown in Fig. 2.2d.

To investigate the formation mechanism of HMSNs, TEM observation was used to show the evolution of the hollow interior. For Na$_2$CO$_3$ etching, a lot of mesopores were present within the solid hollow interior when the Na$_2$CO$_3$

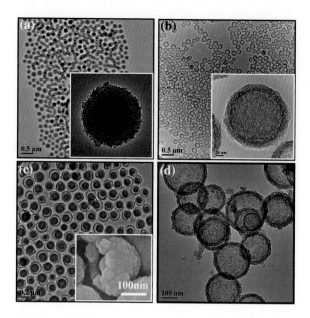

Fig. 2.2 TEM images of sSiO₂@mSiO₂ (**a**), HMSNs obtained by Na₂CO₃ etching (**b**), rattle-type HMSNs obtained by ammonium etching (**c**) and HMSNs obtained by Na₂CO₃ etching. Reproduced with permission from Ref. [28]. © 2010, American Chemical Society

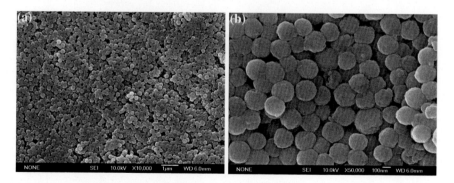

Fig. 2.3 SEM images of homogeneous rattle-type mesoporous silica spheres achieved by treating sSiO₂@mSiO₂ in 0.12 M ammonia solution at 150 °C for 24 h at different magnifications

concentration was decreased (Fig. 2.4). For ammonia etching, the low-etchant concentration induced the formation of hollow interior between the solid core and mesoporous shell (Fig. 2.2c). Therefore, the evolution of the hollow interior in different etchants and etching processes varied significantly.

Based on the above results, we proposed a "structural difference-based selective etching" (SDSA) strategy to synthesize HMSNs (Fig. 2.5). After coating a mesoporous silica layer onto the surface of SiO₂ nanoparticles, the condensation degree of solid SiO₂ core is significantly lower than that of mesoporous

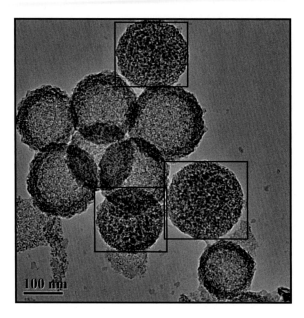

Fig. 2.4 Hollow mesoporous silica spheres obtained by treating sSiO$_2$@mSiO$_2$ in 0.2 M Na$_2$CO$_3$ solution at 80 °C for 0.5 h

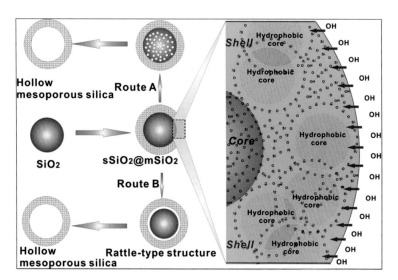

Fig. 2.5 The formation schematics of hollow/rattle-type mesoporous silica spheres (*left*) and the microscopic structure illustration (*right*). Reproduced with permission from Ref. [28]. © 2010, American Chemical Society

silica layer using C$_{18}$TMS as the pore-making agent. Thus, the stability of SiO$_2$ core is lower than that of mesoporous silica shell, by which the SiO$_2$ core can be selectively etched away while the mesoporous silica shell keeps intact. The

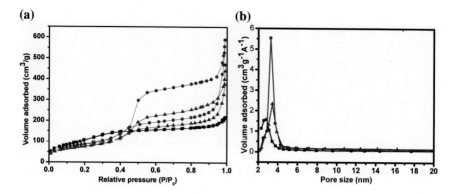

Fig. 2.6 N$_2$ adsorption–desorption isotherms (**a**) and pore size distributions (**b**) of sSiO$_2$@mSiO$_2$ (■), rattle-type mesoporous silica (●) and HMSs (▲) obtained by treating in 0.12 and 0.24 M ammonium solution for 24 h, respectively. Reproduced with permission from Ref. [28]. © 2010, American Chemical Society

hydrophobic part of C$_{18}$TMS self-assembles with hydrolyzed/condensed silica precursors to form worm-like mesopores. When the low Na$_2$CO$_3$ concentration was (0.2 M) used, the SiO$_2$ core could form a lot of mesopores, and further etching could completely remove the core. Under the ammonia etching at high temperature, the less condensed solid S$_i$O$_2$ core condenses further to make the solid silica core difficult to be etched away. Thus, the etching process was from the outside part to the inner part. The rattle-type hollow nanostructure can be formed by this process. Further increase of ammonia concentration can generate the entire hollow nanostructure.

The well-defined mesoporous structure of HMSNs was characterized by typical N$_2$ adsorption–desorption technique. The isotherms of sSiO$_2$@mSiO$_2$, rattle-type HMSNs, and HMSNs exhibit the typical Langmuir IV hysteresis (Fig. 2.6a). Compared to initial sSiO$_2$@mSiO$_2$ and HMSNs, the rattle-type HMSNs show a large hysteresis loop, which indicates that the ink bottle-type mesopores are present within the shell. According to the calculation of the desorption branch of N$_2$ isotherm by BJH method, the average mesopore sizes of rattle-type and hollow mesoporous silica were 3.2 nm and 3.4 nm, respectively (Fig. 2.6b). The enlarged mesopore size was due to the slight etching of the framework of the shell during the chemical etching process. Such an etching process could cause the significant increase of pore volume from 0.33 cm^3/g (sSiO$_2$@mSiO$_2$) to 0.66 cm^3/g (rattle-type HMSNs) due to the formation of large hollow cavity within HMSNs.

The particle size of HMSNs was controlled by choosing the initial SiO$_2$ templates with different particulate sizes. The mature Stöber method facilitates the fabrication of SiO$_2$ templates. As shown in Fig. 2.7, the particle sizes of HMSNs were adjusted to be about 60 nm (Fig. 2.7a), 180 nm (Fig. 2.7b), and 360 nm (Fig. 2.7c). More precise controlling of the particle size can be achieved by choosing different sized SiO$_2$ cores, which is also one of the specific features of hard-templating method to easily control the particle size of hollow nanoparticles.

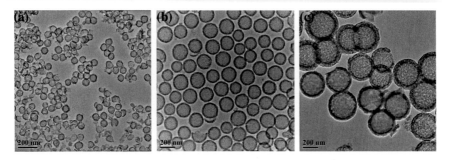

Fig. 2.7 TEM images of HMSNs with different particle sizes: **a** 60, **b** 180 and **c** 360 nm

2.3.2 Synthesis of Multifunctional M@mSiO₂ Nanorattles

Various inorganic functional nanocrystals could be coated with SiO_2 layer by either Stöber method (for hydrophilic nanoparticles) or reversed-phase microemulsion method (for hydrophobic nanoparticles), which can change the surface status of nanocrystals and facilitate their further applications [22−26]. This research sub-area has become relatively mature. It was considered that the formation of solid SiO_2 layer and mesoporous SiO_2 layer was both based on the traditional sol-gel chemical procedure. Therefore, it is easy to coat a mesoporous silica layer onto the surface of solid SiO_2 layer to form $M@SiO_2@mSiO_2$ multilayer composite structure (M: inorganic nanocrystals). Based on the above-mentioned SDSE method, the middle solid SiO_2 layer of $M@SiO_2@mSiO_2$ could be selectively etched away to form $M@mSiO_2$ with large hollow cavity between the core and shell (Fig. 2.8a).

To demonstrate the versatility of SDSE strategy, we employed Au nanoparticles as the functional core to fabricate rattle-type $Au@mSiO_2$ nanoparticles. Au nanoparticles were initially synthesized by a sodium citrate reduction method, followed by coating a dense SiO_2 layer onto the surface of Au nanoparticles ($Au@SiO_2$). Furthermore, a mesoporous silica layer was deposited onto the surface of $Au@SiO_2$ to form $Au@SiO_2@mSiO_2$ composites. The middle solid SiO_2 layer was selectively etched away with the treatment in Na_2CO_3 solution (0.05 M, 80 °C) for 10 min. The triple-layer structured $Au@SiO_2@mSiO_2$ nanoparticles were revealed by the contrast difference in TEM image (Fig. 2.8b). The middle SiO_2 layer could be completely removed to form the rattle-type hollow structure (Fig. 2.8c). The as-prepared $Au@mSiO_2$ exhibited the similar ink bottle-type mesoporous structure with the surface area of 297 m^2/g, pore volume of 0.48 cm^3/g, and average pore size of 4.6 nm (Fig. 2.9a and b). The presence of Au nanocrystals was further demonstrated by X-ray diffraction patter (Fig. 2.9d, JCPDS No. 04-0784). The maximum adsorption peak of $Au@SiO_2@mSiO_2$ at 536 nm showed a 10 nm red shift compared to initial Au nanoparticles (526 nm), and $Au@mSiO_2$ (532 nm) showed a 4 nm blue shift compared to that of $Au@SiO_2@mSiO_2$ (Fig. 2.9c). Such a change in the maximum adsorption peak is due to the variations of the local refractive index of the surrounding medium [27].

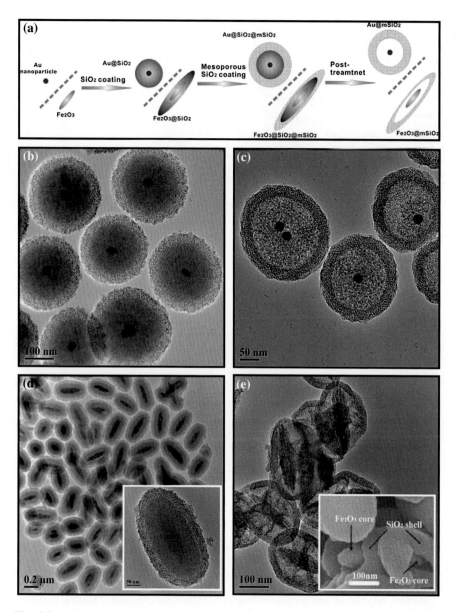

Fig. 2.8 a: Schematic illustration of the synthetic procedures of heterogeneous rattle-type mesoporous nanostructures with inorganic nanocrystals (e.g., spherical Au and ellipsoidal Fe$_2$O$_3$ nanoparticles) as the core and mesoporous silica as the shell; TEM images of Au@SiO$_2$@mSiO$_2$ (**b**), rattle-type Au@mSiO$_2$ (**c**), ellipsoidal Fe$_2$O$_3$@SiO$_2$@mSiO$_2$ (**d** and *inset* picture), rattle-type Fe$_2$O$_3$@mSiO$_2$ (**e**, *inset* SEM image of selected broken ellipsoids). Reproduced with permission from Ref. [28]. © 2010, American Chemical Society

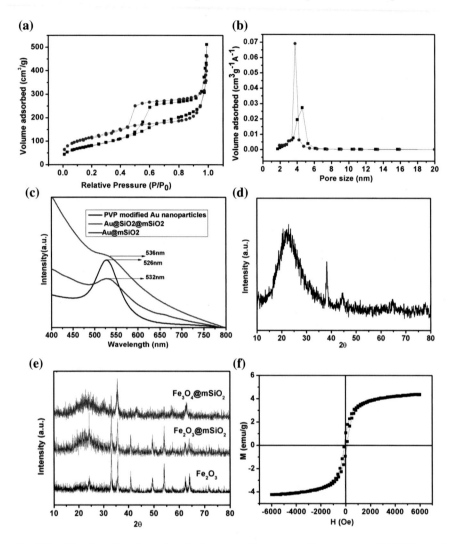

Fig. 2.9 **a** N_2 adsorption–desorption isotherms and **b** corresponding pore size distributions of Au@mSiO$_2$ (■) and Fe$_2$O$_3$@mSiO$_2$ (●); **c** UV-vis spectra of PVP-modified Au nanoparticles, Au@SiO$_2$@mSiO$_2$, and Au@mSiO$_2$; **d** XRD pattern of Au@mSiO$_2$; **e** XRD patterns of ellipsoidal Fe$_2$O$_3$ and Fe$_2$O$_3$@mSiO$_2$ and Fe$_3$O$_4$@mSiO$_2$; **f** Magnetic properties of Fe$_3$O$_4$@mSiO$_2$ after H$_2$ reduction. Reproduced with permission from Ref. [28]. © 2010, American Chemical Society

In order to further reveal that the composition, nanostructure and morphology of M@mSiO$_2$ could be easily controlled, we chose ellipsoidal Fe$_2$O$_3$ as another example to synthesize rattle-type Fe$_2$O$_3$@mSiO$_2$. Monodispersed ellipsoidal Fe$_2$O$_3$ was synthesized by a typical hydrothermal synthesis. After sequentially coating a dense SiO$_2$ layer and a mesoporous SiO$_2$ layer onto the surface, the as-synthesized $Fe_2O_3@SiO_2@mSiO_2$ was treated in ammonia solution to remove the middle solid SiO_2 layer. As shown in Fig. 2.8d and e, the triple-layer structured $Fe_2O_3@SiO_2@mSiO_2$ could be clearly distinguished by the contrast differences. The middle SiO_2 layer could be completely etched away by ammonia solution, further demonstrating the versatility of SDSE strategy. Importantly, the Fe_2O_3 core could be converted to magnetic Fe_3O_4 nanocrystal, forming $Fe_3O_4@mSiO_2$ nano-rattles. Similar to $Au@mSiO_2$, the obtained $Fe_2O_3@mSiO_2$ also showed the ink bottle-type mesoporous structure with the surface area of 427 m^2/g, pore volume of 0.49 cm^3/g, and pore size of 3.8 nm (Fig. 2.9a and b). The phase change of Fe_2O_3 to Fe_3O_4 was demonstrated by X-ray diffraction patterns (Fig. 2.9e). The magnetic $Fe_3O_4@SiO_2@mSiO_2$ nanorattles possess the saturation magnetization of 4.36 emu/g, which show the high-potential applications in T_2-weighted magnetic resonance imaging, magnetic-targeted drug delivery, and magnetic hyperthermia.

2.3.3 HMSNs for Anticancer Drug Delivery

Based on the successful fabrication of HMSNs, we further evaluated their performance in drug delivery. The hemolytic effect of HMSNs was first assessed. As shown in Fig. 2.10a, HMSNs caused the negligible hemolytic effect against red blood cells (RBCs) at the concentration of 0–200 μg/mL. According to the UV-vis test of the quantitative hemolytic percentage at the wavelength of 541 nm, the hemolytic percentage of HMSNs at the high concentration of 200 μg/mL was only 7.37 %. Such a low hemolysis of HMSNs guarantees the safe intravenous administration of HMSNs for drug delivery.

The drug-loading capacity of HMSNs was evaluated by using doxorubicin (DOX) as the model drug. It was found that the DOX-loading efficiency could reach 98 % when relatively large amount of HMSNs was used (50 mg, Fig. 2.10b). To investigate the maximum drug-loading capability of HMSNs, the adopted amount of HMSNs was reduced. The drug-loading amount could reach as high as 1222 mg/g. Such a high drug-loading capacity was attributed to the contribution of large hollow interior, which leaves more room for drug molecules. The therapeutic efficiency of DOX-loaded HMSNs was assessed against MCF-7 breast cancer cells. As shown in Fig. 2.10c and d, HMSNs themselves exhibited low cytotoxicities, indicating their high biocompatibility. DOX-loaded HMSNs showed enhanced cytotoxicity compared to free DOX. Such an enhanced therapeutic efficiency was due to the DOX delivery mediated by HMSNs, which could enter the cancer cells via endocytosis and release the loaded DOX within the cancer cells. Based on the above results, it can be concluded that HMSNs possess high biocompatibility and drug-loading capacity. When HMSNs are used as the DOX carrier, they show substantially improved therapeutic efficiency compared to free DOX drug.

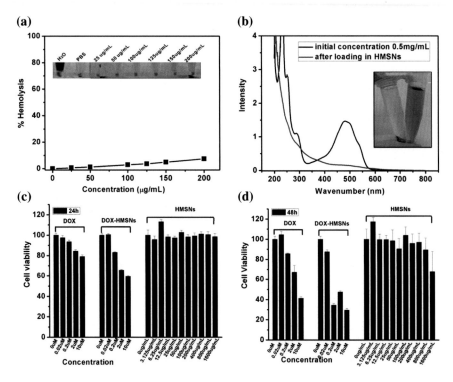

Fig. 2.10 a Hemolysis assay for HMSNs, using water as a positive control and PBS as a negative control (*left*). The HMSNs were suspended at different concentrations (*right*). The mixtures were centrifuged to detect the presence of hemoglobin in the supernatant visually (*inset* picture); **b** UV-vis absorbance spectra of DOX solutions before and after interaction with HMSNs (*inset* digital picture of DOX solution before (*right*) and after interaction (*left*) with HMSNs); **c** and **d** Cell viabilities of free DOX, DOX-loaded HMSNs, and HMSNs at different concentrations and time durations of incubation (**c** 24 h, **d** 48 h). Reproduced with permission from Ref. [28]. © 2010, American Chemical Society

2.4 Conclusions

This chapter developed a novel SDSE strategy to prepare highly dispersed HMSNs with controlled crucial structural parameters. Furthermore, this method was extended to synthesize multifunctional $M@SiO_2$ (M = Au, Fe_2O_3 and Fe_3O_4) hollow nanorattles. The hemolytic effect, cytotoxicity, drug-loading capacity, and therapeutic efficiency of HMSNs were also systematically evaluated. The specific conclusions are listed as follows:

(1)   Based on FTIR and ^{29}Si MAS NMR results, it can be concluded that traditional Stöber-based solid SiO_2 nanoparticles have low condensation degree of silicate framework compared to mesoporous silica nanoparticles templated by surfactants. Based on this chemical mechanism, SDSE method can be developed for the fabrication of HMSNs.

(2) The evolutions of hollow interior of HMSNs by different methods are also substantially different. Chemical etching by Na_2CO_3 initially generates a lot of mesopores within the solid SiO_2 core and further forms the entire hollow interior. Comparatively, etching in ammonia solution initially generates the rattle-type structure and further etches the solid SiO_2 core from the outside part to the inner part.

(3) Such a SDSE strategy can be extended to fabricate various functional $M@mSiO_2$ nanorattles with inorganic nanocrystals as the core, mesoporous silica as the shell, and large hollow cavity in between. In this chapter, three representative nanorattles ($Au@mSiO_2$, $Fe_2O_3@mSiO_2$, and $Fe_3O_4@mSiO_2$) were successfully synthesized by SDSE method.

(4) The particulate sizes of HMSNs could be precisely controlled by choosing the solid SiO_2 core with different sizes. In this chapter, we successfully synthesize HMSNs with the particle sizes of about 60, 180, and 360 nm.

(5) The obtained HMSNs possess high blood compatibility and low cytotoxicity. In addition, HMSNs show high drug (DOX)-loading capacity of as high as 1222 mg/g. Importantly, the therapeutic efficiency of DOX-loaded HMSNs is much higher than free drug.

References

1. LaVan DA, McGuire T, Langer R (2003) Small-scale systems for in vivo drug delivery. Nat Biotechnol 21(10):1184–1191
2. Ashley CE, Carnes EC, Phillips GK, Padilla D, Durfee PN, Brown PA, Hanna TN, Liu JW, Phillips B, Carter MB, Carroll NJ, Jiang XM, Dunphy DR, Willman CL, Petsev DN, Evans DG, Parikh AN, Chackerian B, Wharton W, Peabody DS, Brinker CJ (2011) The targeted delivery of multicomponent cargos to cancer cells by nanoporous particle-supported lipid bilayers. Nat Mater 10(5):389–397
3. Peer D, Karp JM, Hong S, FaroKhzad OC, Margalit R, Langer R (2007) Nanocarriers as an emerging platform for cancer therapy. Nat Nanotechnol 2(12):751–760
4. Slowing II, Vivero-Escoto JL, Wu CW, Lin VSY (2008) Mesoporous silica nanoparticles as controlled release drug delivery and gene transfection carriers. Adv Drug Deliv Rev 60(11):1278–1288
5. Slowing II, Trewyn BG, Giri S, Lin VSY (2007) Mesoporous silica nanoparticles for drug delivery and biosensing applications. Adv Funct Mater 17(8):1225–1236
6. Chen Y, Chen H, Shi J (2013) In Vivo Bio-Safety Evaluations and Diagnostic/Therapeutic Applications of Chemically Designed Mesoporous Silica Nanoparticles. Adv Mater 25(23):3144–3176
7. Tarn D, Ashley CE, Xue M, Carnes EC, Zink JI, Brinker CJ (2013) Mesoporous silica nanoparticle nanocarriers: biofunctionality and biocompatibility. Acc Chem Res 46(3):792–801
8. Tang FQ, Li LL, Chen D (2012) Mesoporous silica nanoparticles: synthesis. Biocompat Drug Deliv Adv. Mater 24(12):1504–1534
9. Huang XL, Li LL, Liu TL, Hao NJ, Liu HY, Chen D, Tang FQ (2011) The shape effect of mesoporous silica nanoparticles on biodistribution, clearance, and biocompatibility in vivo. ACS Nano 5(7):5390–5399
10. Chung TH, Wu SH, Yao M, Lu CW, Lin YS, Hung Y, Mou CY, Chen YC, Huang DM (2007) The effect of surface charge on the uptake and biological function of mesoporous silica nanoparticles 3T3-L1 cells and human mesenchymal stem cells. Biomaterials 28(19):2959–2966

11. Lu F, Wu SH, Hung Y, Mou CY (2009) Size effect on cell uptake in well-suspended, uniform mesoporous silica nanoparticles. Small 5(12):1408–1413
12. He QJ, Zhang ZW, Gao Y, Shi JL, Li YP (2009) Intracellular localization and cytotoxicity of spherical mesoporous silica nano- and microparticles. Small 5(23):2722–2729
13. He QJ, Zhang ZW, Gao F, Li YP, Shi JL (2011) In vivo biodistribution and urinary excretion of mesoporous silica nanoparticles: effects of particle size and PEGylation. Small 7(2):271–280
14. Zhao WR, Chen HR, Li YS, Li L, Lang MD, Shi JL (2008) Uniform rattle-type hollow magnetic mesoporous spheres as drug delivery carriers and their sustained-release property. Adv Funct Mater 18(18):2780–2788
15. Zhu YF, Shi JL, Shen WH, Dong XP, Feng JW, Ruan ML, Li YS (2005) Stimuli-responsive controlled drug release from a hollow mesoporous silica sphere/polyelectrolyte multilayer core-shell structure. Angew Chem-Int Edit 44(32):5083–5087
16. Zhao WR, Lang MD, Li YS, Li L, Shi JL (2009) Fabrication of uniform hollow mesoporous silica spheres and ellipsoids of tunable size through a facile hard-templating route. J Mater Chem 19(18):2778–2783
17. Caruso F, Caruso RA, Mohwald H (1998) Nanoengineering of inorganic and hybrid hollow spheres by colloidal templating. Science 282(5391):1111–1114
18. Li YS, Shi JL, Hua ZL, Chen HR, Ruan ML, Yan DS (2003) Hollow spheres of mesoporous aluminosilicate with a three-dimensional pore network and extraordinarily high hydrothermal stability. Nano Lett 3(5):609–612
19. Zhu YF, Shi JL, Chen HR, Shen WH, Dong XP (2005) A facile method to synthesize novel hollow mesoporous silica spheres and advanced storage property. Microporous Mesoporous Mater 84(1–3):218–222
20. Lou XW, Archer LA, Yang ZC (2008) Hollow Micro-/Nanostructures: Synthesis and Applications. Adv Mater 20(21):3987–4019
21. Stober W, Fink A, Bohn E (1968) Controlled growth of monodisperse silica spheres in micron size range. J Colloid Interface Sci 26(1):62–000
22. Grzelczak M, Correa-Duarte MA, Liz-Marzan LM (2006) Carbon nanotubes encapsulated in wormlike hollow silica shells. Small 2(10):1174–1177
23. Roca M, Haes AJ (2008) Silica-void-gold nanoparticles: temporally stable surf ace-enhanced raman scattering substrates. J Am Chem Soc 130(43):14273–14279
24. Giersig M, Ung T, LizMarzan LM, Mulvaney P (1997) Direct observation of chemical reactions in silica-coated gold and silver nanoparticles. Adv Mater 9(7):570
25. Zhu YF, Kockrick E, Ikoma T, Hanagata N, Kaskel S (2009) An efficient route to rattle-type $Fe_3O_4@SiO_2$ hollow mesoporous spheres using colloidal carbon spheres templates. Chem Mater 21(12):2547–2553
26. Yi DK, Lee SS, Papaefthymiou GC, Ying JY (2006) Nanoparticle architectures templated by SiO_2/Fe_2O_3 nanocomposites. Chem Mater 18(3):614–619
27. LizMarzan LM, Giersig M, Mulvaney P (1996) Synthesis of nanosized gold-silica core-shell particles. Langmuir 12(18):4329–4335
28. Chen Y, Chen HR, Guo LM, He QJ, Chen F, Zhou J, Feng JW, Shi JL (2010) Hollow/rattle-type mesoporous nanostructures by a structural difference-based selective etching strategy. ACS Nano 4(1):529–539

Chapter 3
Multifunctional Mesoporous Silica Nanoparticles for Theranostics of Cancer

3.1 Introduction

The commercial drug capsules effectively encapsulate high amounts of drugs into the large hollow interior. By gradual degradation of shell materials, the drugs can be released from the interior. This drug delivery mode has been widely accepted for oral drug administration. Because of the large particle sizes of commercial capsules (millimeter or centimeter), they are impossible to be injected by intravenous administration. Thus, it is highly desirable to reduce the sizes of capsules into micro/nano-size range to meet the requirements of intravenous injection. Recently developed nanotechnology can effectively solve this critical issue.

With the development of nanosynthetic chemistry, various organic, inorganic, and even organic/inorganic hybrid micro/nanocapsules have been successfully constructed. The mostly developed and explored capsules are the organic microcapsules obtained by layer-by-layer self-assembly, which have been successfully employed for the therapy of tumor and HIV [1–8]. However, the organic materials suffer from the low stability, which easily collapse within the body, causing the explosive release of encapsulated drugs [1, 9–13]. Thus, they are difficult to achieve the sustained release of drugs for chemotherapy. Comparatively, inorganic nanocapsules with well-defined porous structures are featured with high chemical/ thermal stability, sustained drug-releasing behavior, and abundant chemical groups for further modifications, which have attracted the great attention of researchers. To date, various inorganic nanocapsules with different compositions and nanostructures have been successfully fabricated, including mesoporous silica, mesoporous carbon, magnetic Fe_3O_4, $CaCO_3$, fluorescent nanoparticles, etc., [14, 15].

In addition, elaborate multifunctionalization of nanocapsules can obtain a unique kind of multifunctional drug delivery nanosystems. Such a multifunctionalization process can endow the nanocapsules with the function of molecular imaging [16–18]. The most adopted method for multifunctionalization is to introduce various

© Springer-Verlag Berlin Heidelberg 2016
Y. Chen, *Design, Synthesis, Multifunctionalization and Biomedical Applications of Multifunctional Mesoporous Silica-Based Drug Delivery Nanosystems*, Springer Theses, DOI 10.1007/978-3-662-48622-1_3

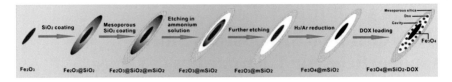

Fig. 3.1   Schematic representation for the preparation of Fe_3O_4@mSiO_2 nanoparticles. Reproduced with permission from Ref. [21]. © 2010, American Chemical Society

functional nanocrystals with magnetic, fluorescent, and thermal properties, such as Au, Ag, quantum dots (QDs), and magnetic Fe_3O_4. Organic fluorescent molecules, paramagnetic centers or targeted molecules/antibodies can also be integrated into the nanocapsules toward multifunctionalization. However, it is difficult to concurrently endow the nanocapsules with the functions of molecular imaging and high drug-loading capacity. This multifunctionalization strategy within single nanocarrier is of great significance to simultaneously realize the diagnosis and therapy of diseases.

In Chap. 2, we have successfully developed a "structural difference-based selective etching" (SDSE) strategy to synthesize HMSNs with unique large hollow interior and well-defined mesoporous structure. The creation of large hollow interior can efficiently enhance the drug-loading capacity of HMSNs. In this chapter, we will continue to synthesize hollow mesoporous nanostructures to endow them with the capabilities of concurrent enhanced drug-loading capacity and molecular imaging. This design strategy will create the nanostructures with Fe_2O_3, Fe_3O_4, and Au nanocrystals as the inner core, mesoporous silica as the shell and large hollow interior between the core and shell. For Fe_3O_4@mSiO_2 rattle-type nanoparticles (Fig. 3.1), ellipsoidal Fe_2O_3 was chosen as the inner core, which was further coated by a solid SiO_2 layer (Fe_2O_3@SiO_2). The ellipsoidal morphology was adopted because the nanoparticles with high aspect ratio were reported to enhance the endocytosis capability of nanoparticles. Then, another mesoporous silica layer templated by C_{18}TMS was coated onto the surface of Fe_2O_3@SiO_2 to form Fe_2O_3@SiO_2@mSiO_2. After further etching the middle SiO_2 layer in ammonia solution by SDSE strategy, the large hollow interior could be generated between Fe_2O_3 core and mesoporous SiO_2 shell. Finally, the Fe_2O_3 core was reduced under H_2/Ar atmosphere to form magnetic Fe_3O_4 core. This chapter systematically investigated the material structure, intracellular endocytosis/location, cytotoxicity, and blood compatibility. In addition, the performance of Fe_3O_4@mSiO_2 for in vitro and in vivo MR imaging was investigated. Doxorubicin (DOX) was selected as the model drug to be encapsulated into Fe_3O_4@mSiO_2 for enhanced chemotherapy.

3.2 Experimental Section

3.2.1 Synthesis of Fe_3O_4@mSiO_2

The synthetic procedure for Fe_3O_4@mSiO_2 was similar to Chap. 2. The procedure was slightly changed to synthesize the nanocapsules with high dispersity. The as-synthesized $Fe_2O_3@SiO_2@mSiO_2$ was divided into two parts, and each part was dispersed into water solution (50 mL) by mild ultrasound treatment. Another ammonia solution (7 mL) was added into above dispersion. The solution was transferred into an autoclave (100 mL volume), which was treated at 150 °C for different durations (4, 12 and 24 h). The following treatment was the same as the procedure described in Chap. 2.

3.2.2 Synthesis of Gd-Si-DPTA-Au@mSiO₂

$Au@mSiO_2$ nanorattles were initially synthesized based on the procedure described in Chap. 2. Gd-Si-DTPA was synthesized according to the following procedures [19]. Diethylenetriamine pentaacetic acid dianhydride (0.5 g) was dissolved in anhydrous pyridine (11 mL) under nitrogen flow, followed by adding 3-Aminopropyltriethoxysilane (APTES, 0.685 g) dropwise. The mixture was stirred at room temperature for 24 h under the protection of nitrogen. The product was precipitated by hexane and collected by centrifugation, which was further washed by hexanes and dried under vacuum (Si-DTPA). The Gd-Si-DTPA was synthesized by dissolving as-synthesized Si-DTPA into NaOH solution (0.6 mL, 1.0 mol/L) by mild ultrasound treatment. Then, $GdCl_3$ aqueous solution (0.4 mL, 0.5 mol/L) was added into above solution, which was incubated for 6 h. The final solution was adjusted to 1 mL to obtain Gd-Si-DTPA for further use.

To prepare $Gd-Si-DTPA-Au@mSiO_2$, the as-synthesized $Au@mSiO_2$ nanorattles were dispersed into water (10 mL) by mild ultrasound treatment, followed by adding Gd-Si-DPTA (500 μL), which was stirred at room temperature for 24 h. The sample were collected by centrifugation and washed by water for three times, which were dried under vacuum at room temperature.

3.2.3 Blood Compatibility of Fe₃O₄@mSiO₂

(A) Hemolytic effect

The evaluation of $Fe_3O_4@mSiO_2$ hemolytic effect was the same as the evaluation procedures of HMSNs as described in Chap. 2 [20].

(B) Coagulation effect

The blood plasma was initially separated from blood for further assessment. $Fe_3O_4@mSiO_2$ nanoparticles were dispersed into PBS at different concentrations (25, 50, 100, 200, and 500 μg/mL), which was then added into fresh human blood plasma (kindly provided by Shanghai Blood Center) for 10 min. After centrifugation, the upper supernatants were obtained for testing on a ACL^{TM} 7000 blood coagulation analyzer according to the standard procedure of HemosIL^{TM} kit (Instrumentation Laboratory Company-Lexington, MA 02421-3125 (USA)). Based on the evaluation procedure, the levels of prothrombin time (PT) and thromboplastin time (APTT) could be obtained.

3.2.4 In Vitro Cytotoxicity of Fe_3O_4@$mSiO_2$ Nanocapsules

In vitro cytotoxicity of Fe_3O_4@$mSiO_2$ was evaluated against different cell lines (MCF-7, HeLa and L929 cells). The cells were initially seeded into 96-well plates at the density of 1×10^4, which were then incubated at the condition of 37 °C and 5 % CO_2 for 24 h. The Fe_3O_4@$mSiO_2$ nanocapsules were dispersed into cell-culturing medium by mild ultrasound treatment at the concentrations of 100, 200, and 400 μg/mL. The culture medium of cells was replaced with Fe_3O_4@$mSiO_2$ solution, which was then co-incubated at 37 °C under 5 % CO_2 for 24 and 48 h. After the co-incubation, the medium was replaced by MTT solution (100 μL, 0.8 mg/mL) and then incubated at 37 °C under 5 % CO_2 for 4 h. DMSO (100 μL) was used to substitute MTT solution, and the absorbance of the solution was tested at the wavelength of 490 nm. The cell viability was expressed as the percentage of the cell viabilities of control cells without any treatment.

3.2.5 Drug-Loading and Anticancer Efficiency

Magnetic Fe_3O_4@$mSiO_2$ nanocapsules were dispersed into DOX PBS solution (5 mL, 0.5 mg/mL), which was stirred for 24 h in the dark. DOX-loaded Fe_3O_4@$mSiO_2$ nanocapsules were collected by centrifugation. To determine the DOX-loading capacity, the supernatant was collected and tested by UV-vis at the wavelength of 480 nm. To test the anticancer efficiency of DOX-loaded Fe_3O_4@$mSiO_2$ nanocapsules, breast cancer MCF-7 cell lines were chosen as the model cells. The evaluation was based on the MTT approach. The evaluation procedure was similar to the MTT process to determine the cytotoxicity of Fe_3O_4@$mSiO_2$ nanocapsules. The differences are the initial cell density (2×10^3 per cell in this case) and the DOX concentrations (0.1, 1, 5, and 20 μg/mL)

3.2.6 CLSM Observations of the Cell Internalization of Fe_3O_4@$mSiO_2$ Nanocapsules

Grafting of FITC into Fe_3O_4@$mSiO_2$ Fluorescein isothiocyanate (FITC) was dispersed into ethanol solution (5 mL), which was pre-dissolved with 3-aminopropyltriethoxysilane (APTES, 100 μL). The mixture was reacted in the dark for 24 h at room temperature. Then, Fe_3O_4@$mSiO_2$ nanocapsules (20 mg) were reacted with FITC-APTES (1 mL ethanol solution) for 24 h. The FITC-grafted Fe_3O_4@$mSiO_2$ nanocapsules were collected by centrifugation, washed by ethanol, and dried at room temperature.
CLSM observation Breast cancer MCF-7 cells were pre-seeded into a 6-well plate with one piece of cover glass at the bottom of each well. Then, the culture

medium was replaced with $Fe_3O_4@mSiO_2$ solution (100 μg/mL) dispersed within cell-culturing medium. After 3 h co-incubation, the culture medium was removed, and the cells were washed by PBS for several times. The cover glass was observed under a laser scanning confocal microscope (FLuoView FV1000, Olympus).

3.2.7 Bio-TEM Observations

MCF-7 cancer cells were initially co-incubated with magnetic $Fe_3O_4@mSiO_2$ nanocapsules at the concentration of 200 μg/mL for 24 h. After co-incubation, the cells were washed by D-hanks and detached by trypsin for 5 min. The cells were collected by centrifugation at 5000 r/min for 2 min. The collected MCF-7 cells were fixed by glutaraldehyde at room temperature, which were further rinsed with PB and dehydrated through a graded ethanol series, and finally cleared with propylene oxide. The cells were then embedded in EPOM812 and polymerized in the oven at 37 °C for 12 h, 45 °C for 12 h, and 60 °C for 48 h. The ultrathin sections of about 70-nm thick were cut by a diamond knife on a Leica UC6 ultramicrotome, which were then transferred to the copper grid. The TEM image was acquired on JEM-1230 electron microcopy.

3.2.8 In Vitro and In Vivo MR Imaging

In vitro MRI experiment was conducted on a 3.0 T clinical MRI instrument (GE Signa 3.0 T). The $Fe_3O_4@mSiO_2$ nanocapsules were dispersed into water solution and the Fe concentration was determined by ICP-AES. The T_2-weighted MRI parameters are described as follows: TR = 4000 ms, Slice = 3.0 mm, TE = 98 ms, echo length = 25 ms.

For in vivo MRI evaluation, the mice tumor xenograft of C57/BL6 melanoma was initially established for assessment. The T_2-weighted in vivo MRI was conducted before and after injection of $Fe_3O_4@mSiO_2$ nanocapsules at the given time intervals (1, 4, and 24 h; concentration: 500 μg/mL). In addition, $Fe_3O_4@mSiO_2$ nanocapsules at the concentrations of 250, 500, and 1000 μg/mL were injected into mice right at the tumor site for MR imaging. The animal procedures were in agreement with the guidelines of the Institutional Animal Care and Use Committee of Chongqing Medical University.

3.2.9 Dark-Field Microscopic Labeling of HeLa Cancer Cells

HeLa cells at the density of about 80 % were pre-seeded in the plate for the co-incubation with Gd-Si-DTPA-grafted $Au@mSiO_2$ nanocapsules at the concentration of 100 μg/mL. After the co-incubation, the cells were washed by D-hanks for three times. The dark-field microscopic images were obtained on Olympus BX51 optical microscopy, using a dark-field imaging accessory.

3.3 Results and Discussion

3.3.1 Synthesis of Characterization of Fe$_3$O$_4$@mSiO$_2$

Rattle-type Fe$_3$O$_4$@mSiO$_2$ with large hollow interior could be fabricated by SDSE strategy. The middle dense silica layer shows the significant hydrolysis/condensation differences compared to outer mesoporous silica layer. The condensation degree of middle silica layer is much lower than that of outer mesoporous silica shell, by which the middle silica layer could be etched away under alkaline environment but the mesoporous silica shell could keep intact. Thus, the large hollow interior could be formed by this unique alkaline etching procedure. From TEM images (Fig. 3.2a–c), it was found that either silica coating or mesoporous silica coating could keep the initial morphology of Fe$_2$O$_3$ template. After further alkaline etching in ammonia solution, the formed large hollow interior could be distinguished by the contrast difference (Fig. 3.2d), demonstrating the feasibility of SDSE strategy. The ellipsoidal morphology of Fe$_3$O$_4$@mSiO$_2$ nanorattles could be observed by SEM observation (Fig. 3.2e and f). Previous report has demonstrated that hydrothermal treatment of Fe$_2$O$_3$@SiO$_2$@mSiO$_2$ could generate the hollow interior within the nanoparticles. The generation of hollow interior was due to the further condensation of silica layer with low condensation degree. The introduction of ammonia solution to increase the pH values could completely remove the middle silica layer, which generated much larger room for the encapsulation of guest molecules. Thus, the loading capacity of as-synthesized nanorattles could be significantly enhanced.

Small-angle X-ray diffraction patterns (Fig. 3.3a) of Fe$_2$O$_3$@mSiO$_2$ and Fe$_3$O$_4$@mSiO$_2$ show no obvious diffraction peaks, indicating that the mesopores are disordered. Such a disordered nature of mesopore is determined by the organosilica C$_{18}$TMS as the pore-making agent. The phase transformation of Fe$_2$O$_3$ to Fe$_3$O$_4$ was demonstrated by the wide-angle X-ray diffraction patterns (Fig. 3.3b). The XRD pattern of Fe$_3$O$_4$@mSiO$_2$ shows the characteristic peak of Fe$_3$O$_4$ nanocrystal, while the representative XRD peaks of Fe$_2$O$_3$ disappear, indicating that the Fe$_2$O$_3$ core was reduced to Fe$_3$O$_4$ under reducing environment. Figure 3.3c shows that as-synthesized Fe$_2$O$_3$@mSiO$_2$ and Fe$_3$O$_4$@mSiO$_2$ could be well dispersed into aqueous solution, and the Fe$_3$O$_4$@mSiO$_2$ nanorattles could be manipulated by external magnetic field.

The evolution of hollow interior was observed by TEM images after different etching durations. As shown in Fig. 3.4a–c, the hollow cavity was initially formed between the solid silica and mesoporous silica, which extended into the interior with the etching time. Finally, the hollow silica layer was completed removed. This formation mechanism of hollow cavity was the same as the fabrication

Fig. 3.2 TEM images
of ellipsoidal Fe_2O_3
(**a**), $Fe_2O_3@SiO_2$ (**b**),
$Fe_2O_3@SiO_2@mSiO_2$ (**c**),
and $Fe_3O_4@mSiO_2$ (**d**);
Secondary electron SEM
image of ellipsoidal Fe_2O_3
(**e**, *inset* SEM image at
high magnification) and
backscattered SEM image
(**f**) of ellipsoidal
$Fe_3O_4@mSiO_2$ nanocapsules
(*inset* purposely selected
backscattered SEM image
of broken nanocapsules
to reveal the hollow
nanostructure). Reproduced
with permission from
Ref. [21]. © 2010, American
Chemical Society

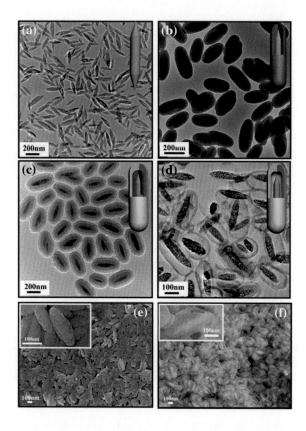

of rattle-type $sSiO_2@mSiO_2$. N_2 adsorption–desorption technique was used to characterize the changes of mesoporous structures before and after chemical etching. It was found that the etched $Fe_3O_4@mSiO_2$ showed much larger hysteresis loop than initial $Fe_3O_4@SiO_2@mSiO_2$ (Fig. 3.5a–b), indicating the formation of ink-in-bottle-type mesoporous structure. The surface area increased from 261 to 318 m^2/g while the pore volume increased from 0.44 to 0.78 cm^3/g after chemical etching. The pore size also increased from initial 2.5 to 3.6 nm. The mechanism of changes on mesoporous parameters was the same as Chap. 2 on the HMSNs. The Si–O–Si bonds within the mesoporous shell were not stable under hydrothermal condition, which could break up to confuse with each other, causing the increase of mesopore sizes (Fig. 3.5c).

3.3.2 Magnetic Fe₃O₄@mSiO₂ for MRI and Anticancer Drug Delivery

The efficient internalization of nanoparticles by cancer cells determines the possibility of drugs to be delivered into cells. To facilitate the observation by confocal

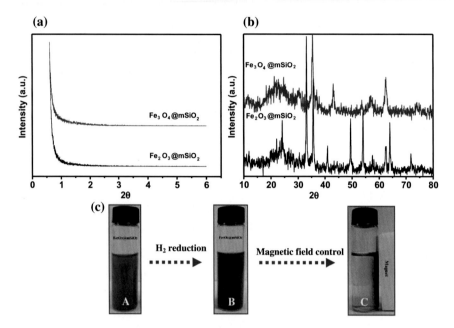

Fig. 3.3 Small-angle (**a**) and wide-angle (**b**) X-ray diffraction patterns of Fe_2O_3@mSiO$_2$ and Fe_3O_4@mSiO$_2$ nanocapsules; (**c**) Digital pictures of Fe_2O_3@mSiO$_2$ (*A*) and Fe_3O_4@mSiO$_2$ (*B*) dispersed in PBS solution, and Fe_3O_4@mSiO$_2$ nanocapsules in PBS solution under magnetic field (*C*). Reproduced with permission from Ref. [21]. © 2010, American Chemical Society

laser scanning microscopy (CLSM), green fluorescein isothiocyanate (FITC) was grafted into Fe_3O_4@mSiO$_2$. After the co-incubation with FITC-Fe_3O_4@mSiO$_2$ nanocapsules, breast cancer MCF-7 cells were observed by CLSM. Figure 3.6a$_1$–a$_3$ shows that the nanocapsules were efficiently endocytosized into MCF-7 cells demonstrated by the presence of large amounts of fluorescent dots within cancer cells. The overlay of the bright-field and fluorescent images further indicates the intracellular location of the nanocapsules. Further bio-TEM characterization reveals the uptake mechanism and intracellular location of Fe_3O_4@mSiO$_2$ nanocapsules. It was found that the nanocapsules were present in the cytoplasm but no nanoparticles were found in the nucleus (Fig. 3.6b$_1$ and b$_2$). The nanocapsules were also found near the cell membrane to form the vesicles (Fig. 3.6b$_3$). Therefore, Fe_3O_4@mSiO$_2$ nanocapsules could be endocytosized into cancer cells and processed in the endosomes/lysosomes and finally located within the cytoplasm of cancer cells.

The magnetic core of Fe_3O_4@mSiO$_2$ could act as the contrast agents for T$_2$-weighted MR imaging. To evaluate the MRI performance, Fe_3O_4@mSiO$_2$ nanocapsules were initially dispersed into aqueous solution for in vitro experiment. It was found in T$_2$ phantom images that the presence of magnetic core could efficiently shorten the T$_2$ relaxation time, indicating that the nanocapsules have

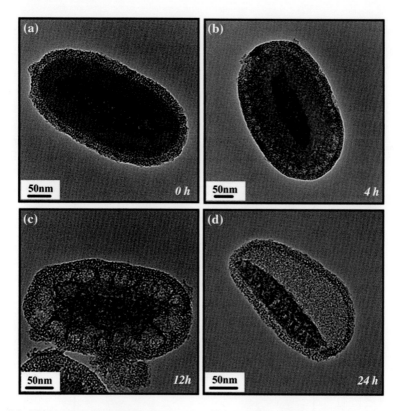

Fig. 3.4 TEM images of magnetic mesoporous composites obtained by etching in an ammonium solution for 0 h (**a**), 4 h (**b**), 12 h (**c**), and 24 h (**d**). Reproduced with permission from ref [21]. © 2010, American Chemical Society

generated the magnetic resonance contrast on transverse proton relaxations-times weighted sequence because of the dipolar interaction of the magnetic moments between the nanocapsules and proton in the water. The calculated relaxation rate r_2 of $Fe_3O_4@mSiO_2$ was 137.8 mM^{-1} s^{-1}. To evaluate the in vivo MRI behavior, the $Fe_3O_4@mSiO_2$ nanocapsules were administrated into mice subcutaneously at different concentrations (250, 500, and 1000 $\mu g/mL$) and time intervals (1, 4, and 24 h), which were further imaged by T_2-weighted MR imaging. It was found that the injection site within tumors showed the obvious darkened area, confirming the imaging capability of the magnetic nanocapsules. In addition, the darkened area became larger as the increase of injected concentration and extended time, indicating the concentration- and time-dependent MR imaging performance of $Fe_3O_4@mSiO_2$ nanocapsules (Fig. 3.6c_1–c_3 and d_1–d_4).

The biocompatibility of $Fe_3O_4@mSiO_2$ nanocapsules determines their further clinical translations. The blood compatibility is of high significance to show the possibility of intravenous administration. The research on the blood compatibility of inorganic multifunctional nanoparticles has not been reported yet. The

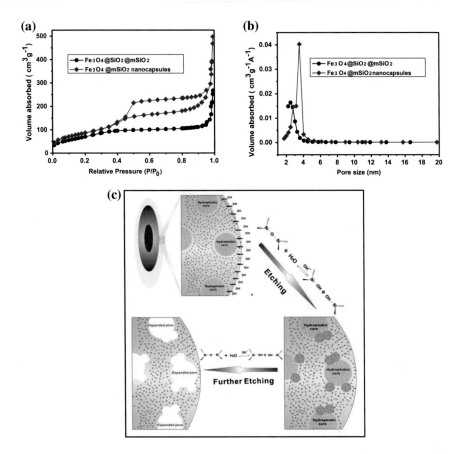

Fig. 3.5 **a** N_2 adsorption–desorption isotherms and **b** corresponding pore size distributions of $Fe_3O_4@SiO_2@mSiO_2$ and $Fe_3O_4@mSiO_2$ nanocapsules after 24 h etching; **c** Schematic representation of the microstructure evolution before, during and after the alkaline etching. Reproduced with permission from Ref. [21]. © 2010, American Chemical Society

hemolytic evaluation was similar to Chap. 2. As shown in Fig. 3.7a, no obvious hemolysis of red blood cells (RBCs) was observed after the co-incubation with $Fe_3O_4@mSiO_2$ nanocapsules at different concentrations. At the concentrations of 300 and 500 µg/mL, the hemolytic percentages were calculated to be only 1.2 and 3.7 %, respectively, much lower than traditional amorphous SiO_2 nanoparticles (44 % hemolytic percentage at the concentration of 100 µg/mL), indicating the low hemolytic effect of $Fe_3O_4@mSiO_2$ nanocapsules.

The coagulation effect of $Fe_3O_4@mSiO_2$ was further evaluated. It was reported that zeolites, mesoporous glasses and MCM41-type mesoporous silica could cause the coagulation because of their large surface are and high absorption volume. It was considered that the coagulation effect must be reduced to as low as possible during the intravenous administration. The fresh isolated plasma was co-incubated

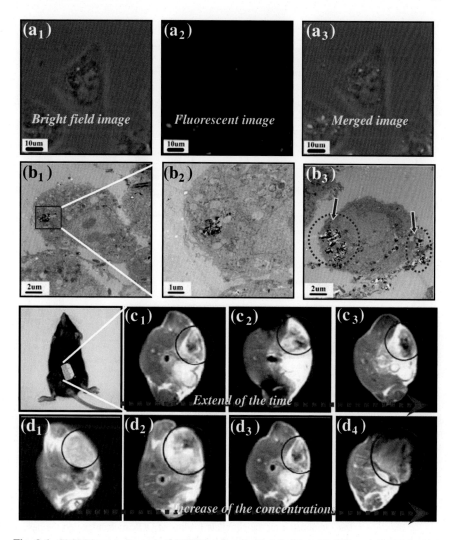

Fig. 3.6 CLSM images (**a₁–a₃**) of MCF-7 cells after incubation with 100 μg/mL FITC-nano-capsules for 3 h; Bio-TEM images (**b₁–b₃**) of MCF-7 cells after incubation with magnetic $Fe_3O_4@mSiO_2$ nanocapsules; In vivo MRI (**c** and **d**) of a tumor-bearing mouse before and after injection of magnetic $Fe_3O_4@mSiO_2$ nanocapsules for different time intervals (**c₁**-1 h; **c₂**-4 h and **c₃**-24 h at 500 μg/mL of $Fe_3O_4@mSiO_2$ nanocapsules) and at different nanocapsule concentrations (**d₁**-control; **d₂**-250 μg/mL; **d₃**-500 μg/mL; **d₄**-1000 μg/mL in 1 h of post-injection). Reproduced with permission from Ref. [21]. © 2010, American Chemical Society

with $Fe_3O_4@mSiO_2$ nanocapsules at different concentrations (25–500 μg/mL) for testing the prothrombin time (PT) and activated partial thromboplastin time (APTT). Figure 3.8a shows the testing procedure and used apparatus during the coagulation evaluation. It was found that the PT and APTT values were all in the normal range (Fig. 3.8b and c), which also showed no significant differences

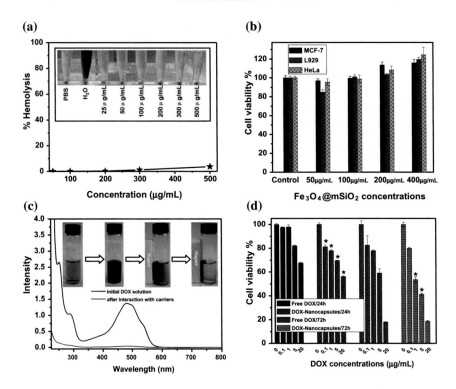

Fig. 3.7 **a** Hemolysis assay for the magnetic nanocapsules (*inset* photographic images for the direct observation of hemolysis by the nanocapsules, using PBS as a negative control and water as positive control (the two tubes on the *left*), and the capsules suspended at different concentrations (the six tubes on the *right*). The red blood cells are red due to the presence of hemoglobin in the RBCs. During the hemolysis assay experiment, hemoglobin will be released into the solution by hemolysis, resulting in visually *red* color in solution; **b** Cell viabilities of the empty nanocapsules against MCF-7 cells at different concentrations for 24 h; **c** UV-vis spectra of DOX before and after interaction with the nanocapsules (*inset*, from the *left* to *right* digital pictures of pure DOX solution, and the nanocapsules added DOX solutions before, after 30 s magnetic field attraction and after complete magnetic field attraction). The color of DOX/PBS solution changed from the *red* to colorless, demonstrating the complete loading of DOX molecules into the nanocapsules; **d** Cell viabilities of free DOX and DOX-loaded Fe_3O_4@mSiO_2 nanocapsules against MCF-7 cells at different DOX concentrations for 24 h and 72 h (*represent significance difference compared with free DOX with the same drug concentration at $P < 0.05$). Reproduced with permission from Ref. [21]. © 2010, American Chemical Society

compared to the control plasma without any treatments. This result gives the direct evidence that Fe_3O_4@mSiO_2 nanocapsules will not cause the coagulation effect. Based on the hemolysis and coagulation evaluations, it could be concluded that the as-synthesized Fe_3O_4@mSiO_2 nanocapsules have high blood compatibility, which meets the requirements of intravenous administration.

The cytotoxicity of Fe_3O_4@mSiO_2 was assessed by the typical MTT method against different cell lines (MCF-7, L929, and HeLa cell lines). It was found that

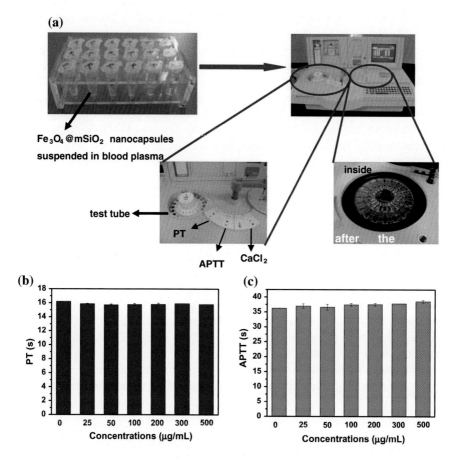

Fig. 3.8 **a** Schematic illustration of the whole procedure for the evaluation of the coagulation effect caused by $Fe_3O_4@mSiO_2$ nanocapsules in PBS. First, $Fe_3O_4@mSiO_2$ nanocapsules (50 µL) with different concentrations (0, 25, 50, 100, 200, 300, and 500 µg/mL) were mixed with the fresh blood plasma (450 µL). After the gentle vortex, the nanoparticles suspended in the plasma were stood still for 10 min. After the centrifugation at 5000 rmp for 5 min, the supernatants were collected and tested on a ACL^{TM} 7000 blood coagulation analyzer using HemosIL^{TM} kit (Instrumentation Laboratory Company-Lexington, MA 02421-3125 (USA)); The kit consists of APTT reagent and calcium chloride was used for coagulation assay; PT (**b**) and APTT (**c**) values of the blood plasma after the exposure to $Fe_3O_4@mSiO_2$ nanocapsules of different concentrations

$Fe_3O_4@mSiO_2$ exhibited no obvious cytotoxicities even at the high concentration of 400 µg/mL (Fig. 3.7b). The $Fe_3O_4@mSiO_2$ nanocapsules were expected to have high drug-loading capacity because of their large hollow interior. Here we chose doxorubicin (DOX) as the anticancer drug to evaluate their drug-loading and delivery performances. The $Fe_3O_4@mSiO_2$ nanocapsules were initially dispersed into DOX PBS solution, which were further collected by centrifugation after 24 h impregnation. The DOX-loading capacity was determined by UV-vis characterizations. As shown in Fig. 3.7c, the characteristic absorption peak at $\lambda = 480$ nm disappeared after the loading process, indicating that the initial DOX was completely encapsulated into the carrier. The drug-loading amount and efficiency of $Fe_3O_4@mSiO_2$ could reach 20, 100 %, respectively. Traditional organic liposomes and micelles have the high drug-loading efficiency but low drug-loading amount. Comparatively, traditional mesoporous SiO_2 nanoparticles possess high drug-loading amount but low encapsulation efficiency. The designed $Fe_3O_4@mSiO_2$ nanocapsules have the large hollow interior, large surface area, and high pore volume. In addition, the electrostatic interaction between positively charged DOX and negatively charged mesopores further enhances the drug-loading capacity. Moreover, the mesoporous structure endows the carrier with sustained drug-releasing feature. Therefore, the achieved $Fe_3O_4@mSiO_2$ nanocapsules could realize the sustained release of drugs to achieve the continuous therapy.

To evaluate the anticancer efficiency of DOX-loaded $Fe_3O_4@mSiO_2$ nanocapsules, the cell viabilities of MCF-7 cancer cells were obtained after the treatment with free DOX and DOX-loaded $Fe_3O_4@mSiO_2$ nanocapsules by traditional MTT method. As shown in Fig. 3.7d, DOX-loaded $Fe_3O_4@mSiO_2$ showed much higher cytotoxicity than that of free DOX, indicating that more DOX could be delivered into cancer cells to induce the cell death. Therefore, the achieved $Fe_3O_4@mSiO_2$ nanocapsules meet the requirements of excellent drug delivery nanosystems. Combined with the T_2-weighted MR imaging performance, it is expected that $Fe_3O_4@mSiO_2$ nanocapsules could act as the promising theranostic agents for diagnostic imaging, therapy, and in situ monitoring of the therapeutic processes.

3.3.3 Synthesis of Gd-Si-DTPA-Grafted Au@mSiO₂ for Biomedical Applications

The SDSE strategy could be further extended to fabricate a series of $M@mSiO_2$ nanostructures. It was considered that Au nanoparticles have been extensive used for biomedical applications. Therefore, we employed Au nanoparticles as the core of $M@mSiO_2$ to fabricate $Au@mSiO_2$ nanocapsules. Furthermore, Gd-Si-DTPA was further grafted into the mesopores using Si-OH groups. As shown in Fig. 3.9, the solid silica core of $Au@SiO_2@mSiO_2$ could be completely removed by selective etching to leave large hollow cavity. After further Gd-Si-DTPA grafting, the mesopores still kept intact. Because of the plasmon resonance effect (Fig. 3.10), the achieved $Au@mSiO_2$ nanocapsules could act as the contrast agents for dark-field cell labeling and T_1-weighted MR imaging.

The capability of Gd-Si-DTPA-grafted $Au@mSiO_2$ nanocapsules for dark-field light-scattering cell labeling was evaluated. As shown in Fig. 3.11b, HeLa cells show large amounts of bright dots intracellularly after the co-incubation with Gd-Si-DTPA@mSiO₂ nanocapsules, which was due to the light-scattering capability

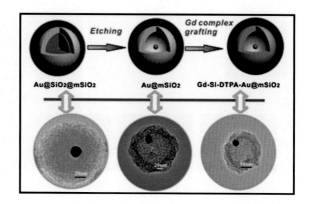

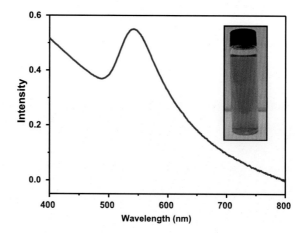

of the Au core. Comparatively, there is no aforementioned phenomenon in the control HeLa cells without any treatment (Fig. 3.11a). This experiment strongly demonstrates the ability of Au@mSiO$_2$ nanocapsules for dark-field light-scattering cell labeling.

Meanwhile, Gd-Si-DTPA-Au@mSiO$_2$ composite nanocapsules could act as the contrast agents for T_1-weighted MR imaging because of the grafted Gd-Si-DPTA (Fig. 3.12a). As shown in Fig. 3.12b, the T_1-weighted MRI signal shows the Gd concentration-dependent enhancement in aqueous solution. The relaxation rate r_1 was calculated to be as high as 7.43 mM^{-1} s^{-1} (Fig. 3.12c), indicating the high performance of Gd-Si-DTPA-Au@mSiO$_2$ nanocapsules for T_1-weighted MR imaging. Such a high performance is due to the high dispersity of Gd-based para-magnetic centers within the mesopores, which facilitates the interaction with water molecules.

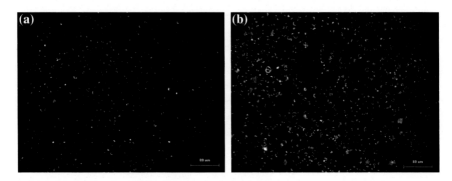

Fig. 3.11 Dark-field optical microscopic images of HeLa cells before (**a**) and after (**b**) incubation with 100 μg/mL Gd-Si-DTPA-grafted Au@mSiO$_2$ nanocapsules. Reproduced with permission from Ref. [21]. © 2010, American Chemical Society

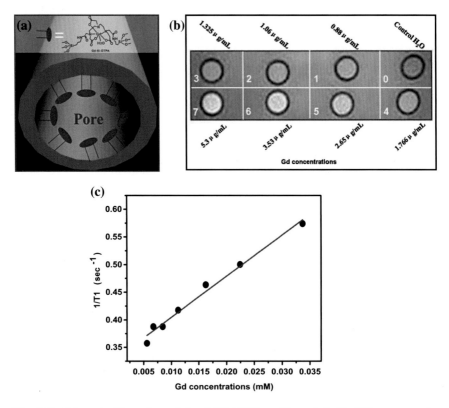

Fig. 3.12 Schematic illustration of the Gd-Si-DTPA grafting of Au@mSiO$_2$ nanocapsules (**a**) and T$_1$-weighted images (**b**) of Gd-Si-DTPA-Au@mSiO$_2$ nanocapsules of different Gd concentrations in water. **c** r_1 relaxation curve of Gd-Si-DTPA-Au@mSiO$_2$ nanocapsules. Reproduced with permission from Ref. [21]. © 2010, American Chemical Society

3.4 Conclusions

Based on SDSE strategy, a series of M@mSiO$_2$ (M = Fe$_2$O$_3$, Fe$_3$O$_4$, Au) composite nanocapsules were successfully fabricated. Their applications in bio-imaging and drug delivery were systematically investigated. The specific conclusions are summarized as follows.

(1) Magnetic Fe$_3$O$_4$ nanoparticles could be successfully introduced into hollow mesoporous silica nanocapsules based on the SDSE strategy, endowing the composite nanocapsules with T$_2$-weighted MR imaging capability.

(2) The fabricated Fe$_3$O$_4$@mSiO$_2$ composite nanocapsules showed excellent blood compatibility, such as low hemolytic and coagulation effects. The formation of large hollow cavity could enhance the drug-loading capacity (DOX, 20 %) and efficiency (nearly 100 %). The DOX delivered mediated by Fe$_3$O$_4$@mSiO$_2$ exhibited enhanced cytotoxicity compared to free DOX drugs.

(3) Gd-Si-DTPA could be successfully grafted into the mesopores of Au@mSiO$_2$ nanocapsules to endow the carrier with T$_1$-weighted MRI ability. The inner Au core could act as the contrast agents for dark-field light-scattering cell labeling. The calculated r_1 for T$_1$-weighted MR imaging was as high as 7.43 mM^{-1} s^{-1}.

References

1. Meier W (2000) Polymer nanocapsules. Chem Soc Rev 29(5):295–303
2. Wang YJ, Bansal V, Zelikin AN, Caruso F (2008) Templated synthesis of single-component polymer capsules and their application in drug delivery. Nano Lett 8(6):1741–1745
3. Qiu XP, Leporatti S, Donath E, Mohwald H (2001) Studies on the drug release properties of polysaccharide multilayers encapsulated ibuprofen microparticles. Langmuir 17(17):5375–5380
4. Wang Y, Angelatos AS, Caruso F (2008) Template synthesis of nanostructured materials via layer-by-layer assembly. Chem Mater 20(3):848–858
5. Pastoriza-Santos I, Scholer B, Caruso F (2001) Core-shell colloids and hollow polyelectrolyte capsules based on diazoresins. Adv Funct Mater 11(2):122–128
6. Yu J, Javier D, Yaseen MA, Nitin N, Richards-Kortum R, Anvari B, Wong MS (2010) Self-assembly synthesis, tumor cell targeting, and photothermal capabilities of antibody-coated indocyanine green nanocapsules. J Am Chem Soc 132(6):1929–1938
7. Sexton A, Whitney PG, Chong SF, Zelikin AN, Johnston APR, De Rose R, Brooks AG, Caruso F, Kent SJ (2009) A protective vaccine delivery system for in vivo T cell stimulation using nanoengineered polymer hydrogel capsules. ACS Nano 3(11):3391–3400
8. Sexton A, Whitney PG, De Rose R, Zelikin AN, Chong S, Johnston AP, Caruso F, Kent SJ (2009) Nanoengineered layer-by-layer capsules as a novel delivery system for HIV vaccines. Retrovirology 6:2
9. van Nostrum CF (2004) Polymeric micelles to deliver photosensitizers for photodynamic therapy. Adv Drug Deliv Rev 56(1):9–16
10. Wang HJ, Zhao PQ, Su WY, Wang S, Liao ZY, Niu RF, Chang J (2010) PLGA/polymeric liposome for targeted drug and gene co-delivery. Biomaterials 31(33):8741–8748
11. Lasic DD, Needham D (1995) The "Stealth" liposome: a prototypical biomaterial. Chem Rev 95(8):2601–2628

12. LaVan DA, McGuire T, Langer R (2003) Small-scale systems for in vivo drug delivery. Nat Biotechnol 21(10):1184–1191
13. Torchilin VP (2005) Recent advances with liposomes as pharmaceutical carriers. Nat Rev Drug Discov 4(2):145–160
14. Cao SW, Zhu YJ, Ma MY, Li L, Zhang L (2008) Hierarchically nanostructured magnetic hollow spheres of Fe_3O_4 and gamma-Fe_2O_3: preparation and potential application in drug delivery. J Phys Chem C 112(6):1851–1856
15. Wei W, Ma GH, Hu G, Yu D, McLeish T, Su ZG, Shen ZY (2008) Preparation of hierarchical hollow $CaCO_3$ particles and the application as anticancer drug carrier. J Am Chem Soc 130(47):15808
16. Lin YS, Wu SH, Hung Y, Chou YH, Chang C, Lin ML, Tsai CP, Mou CY (2006) Multifunctional composite nanoparticles: magnetic, luminescent, and mesoporous. Chem Mater 18(22):5170–5172
17. Shi JL, Chen Y, Chen HR (2013) Progress on the Multifunctional Mesoporous Silica-based Nanotheranostics. J Inorg Mater 28(1):1–11
18. Vivero-Escoto JL, Taylor-Pashow KML, Huxford RC, Huxford RC, Della Rocca J, Okoruwa C, An HY, Lin WL, Lin WB (2011) Multifunctional mesoporous silica nanospheres with cleavable Gd(III) chelates as MRI contrast agents: synthesis, characterization, target-specificity, and renal clearance. Small 7(24):3519–3528
19. Taylor KML, Kim JS, Rieter WJ, An H, Lin WL, Lin WB (2008) Mesoporous silica nanospheres as highly efficient MRI contrast agents. J Am Chem Soc 130(7):2154
20. Slowing II, Wu CW, Vivero-Escoto JL, Lin VSY (2009) Mesoporous silica nanoparticles for reducing hemolytic activity towards mammalian red blood cells. Small 5(1):57–62
21. Chen Y, Chen HR, Zeng DP, Tian YB, Chen F, Feng JW, Shi JL (2010) Core/shell structured hollow mesoporous nanocapsules: a potential platform for simultaneous cell imaging and anticancer drug delivery. ACS Nano 4(10):6001–6013

Chapter 4
Hollow Mesoporous Silica Nanoparticles for Ultrasound-Based Cancer Diagnosis and Therapy

4.1 Introduction

With the development of science/technology and biomedicine, the disease therapy has a fast evolution from harmful surgery to minimally invasive surgical treatment. The development of therapeutic modality substantially enhances the treatment efficiency and concurrently mitigates the side effects. Therefore, the pains of patients can be significantly reduced. The concept of noninvasive therapy is featured with high efficiency, reduced side effects, and low cost, which has become one of the important fields in biomedicine. High-intensity focused ultrasound (HIFU), as the most representative noninvasive therapeutic modality, has found the extensive applications in the ablation of uterine fibroids [1–3]. Typically, the HIFU-based therapeutic mechanism is based on the thermal, mechanical, and ultrasonic-cavitation effects [1–3]. However, it is difficult to ablate the lesions in the deep organs by HIFU because the ultrasound energy is not sufficient enough when it reaches the deep organs. The single increase of ultrasound-emitting power to enhance the energy deposition will cause the tissue damage in ultrasound-propagation path. Therefore, it is highly desirable to develop new strategies to enhance the ultrasound-energy deposition within the lesions accompanying with high therapeutic efficiency and low side effects.

In addition, it is of great significance to precisely determine the targeted lesion tissue before HIFU therapy because the prepositioning of the disease can enhance the HIFU therapeutic efficiency and mitigate the damages to surrounding normal tissues [4, 5]. Currently, two imaging modalities have been successfully integrated into HIFU therapy, including ultrasound imaging (US) and magnetic resonance imaging (MRI). US is convenient, portable, and cost-effective. However, its limited sensitivity and spatial resolution strongly hinder its extensive applications in imaging-guided HIFU ablation. Comparatively, MRI shows much higher spatial and anatomical resolution for HIFU guidance. In addition to the update of

© Springer-Verlag Berlin Heidelberg 2016
Y. Chen, *Design, Synthesis, Multifunctionalization and Biomedical Applications of Multifunctional Mesoporous Silica-Based Drug Delivery Nanosystems*, Springer Theses, DOI 10.1007/978-3-662-48622-1_4

the expensive imaging apparatus, recently developed nanotechnology provides an alternative strategy to solve the critical issues of HIFU therapy, such as efficiency and safety. Previous results have demonstrated that the introduction of organic microbubbles can enhance the HIFU ablation efficiency against tissues [6–11]. However, the large particulate sizes of microbubbles, typically in the range of several micrometers, hinder the microbubbles to enter the tumor tissues across the vascular endothelial gap. Besides, the stability of organic microbubbles is low, which can be easily broken upon HIFU irradiation. Therefore, these microbubbles cannot enhance the HIFU therapeutic efficiency continuously, substantially restricting their extensive clinical applications.

In this chapter, we first synthesized HMSNs based on the developed SDSE strategy, which were further used as the carrier for the encapsulation of perfluorohexane (PFH) organic molecules. The PFH-loaded HMSNs were further employed as the synergistic agents for enhancing the HIFU ablation efficiency. Furthermore, the shell of HMSNs was functionalized for imaging-guided HIFU therapy. Paramagnetic manganese (Mn) centers were uniformly distributed within the mesopores to endow HMSNs with T_1-weighted MRI capability. The obtained multifunctional mesoporous composite nanocapsules (designated as MCNCs) were further used to encapsulate PFH molecules, which can concurrently realize the functions of MRI guidance and HIFU synergistic therapy.

4.2 Experimental Section

4.2.1 Material Synthesis

(A) Synthesis of inorganic mesoporous nanocapsules (designated as IMNCs)
The synthesis of IMNCs was based on SDSE strategy by HF etching of $sSiO_2@mSiO_2$ nanoparticles. The detailed synthetic procedure was similar to Chap. 1.

(B) Synthesis of MCNCs
HMSNs templated by C_{16}TAB were synthesized according to the reported procedure [12]. The as-synthesized HMSNs (50 mg) solution (10 mL) was dispersed into $KMnO_4$ aqueous solution (0.1 M, 10 mL), which was further stirred at 40 °C for 4 h. The product was collected by centrifugation, washed by plenty of water, and dried under vacuum at room temperature. The remaining C_{16}TAB molecules were removed by calcinations (550 °C, 6 h). The final product was treated by H_2/Ar (5 % H_2 volume) at high temperature (500 °C, 4 h).

(C) Synthesis of PFH-IMNCs and PFH-MCNCs
PFH-IMNCs The pre-dried IMNCs (100 mg) were put into a centrifuge tube (15 mL volume), followed by adding PFH dropwise (200 μL). The mouth of the tube was sealed to avid the evaporation of the loaded PFH molecules. PFH-loaded

IMCNs was mildly treated by ultrasound for 30 s in an ice bath. Then, PBS (10 mL) was added into PFH-loaded IMCNs, which was further treated by ultrasound to disperse PFH-loaded IMCNs. Finally, the sample was sealed tightly and stored at room temperature for further use.

PFH-MCNCs The pre-dried MCNCs (300 mg) were put into a centrifuge tube with the volume of 15 mL. The following steps are the same as the loading procedure for PFH-IMNCs. The finial PFH-MCNCs were stored at 4 °C for further use.

4.2.2 In Vitro MRI Evaluation

In vitro MRI evaluation was conducted on a clinical GE Signa 3.0 T MRI apparatus. MCNCs were dispersed into aqueous solution, followed by ICP-AES test to determine Mn concentration. The employed pulse sequence was T_1-weighted FR-FSE sequence. The detailed parameters are described as follows: TR = 1000, 2000, 3000, and 4000, Slice = 3.0 mm, Space = 0.5 mm, Fov = 20, Phase fov = 0.8, Freq × Phase = 384×256, Nex = 2, ETL = 2. The used T_2-weighted sequence was FRFSE-XL sequence with the detailed parameters are Space = 0.5 mm, FOV = 14, TR = 2000, TE = 105, ETL = 16, Freq × Phase = 256 × 192 and Slice = 2.0 mm.

4.2.3 Ex Vivo Evaluation Toward the HIFU Synergistic Effect of IMNCs, PFH-IMNCs, MCNCs, and PFH-MCNCs

Degassed bovine livers were used as the model tissue to ex vivo evaluate the HIFU synergistic effect. The used apparatus is JC-1-type HIFU tumor therapeutic system, which was developed by Chongqing Medial University. The frequencies for therapy and imaging are 3.5 and 1.1 MHz, respectively. Typically, the degassed bovine livers were cut into a cubic shape and put into a tank filled with degassed water. The syringes (1 mL volume) filled with PBS, IMNCs, PFH-IMNCs, and PFH-MCNCs were inset into the bovine liver, respectively. Ultrasound imaging was used to monitor the injection site. After the quick injection of different agents (200 µL), HIFU was directly acted on the injection site (150 W/cm^2, 5 s; 250 W/cm^2, 5 s). The used concentration of MCNCs was 30 mg/mL. Ultrasonic echo-signal was recorded by the software GrayVal 1.0 (Chongqing Haifu Technology Company, Chongqing, P. R. China). After the HIFU irradiation, the coagulated tissue volume in degassed bovine was calculated by the following equation: $V = \pi/6 \times L_{max} \times W_{max}^2$ (L_{max}: the maximum length of coagulated tissue, W_{max}: the maximum width of coagulated tissue). Each test was repeated for three times to obtain the average values of different values.

4.2.4 CLSM Observation of Intracellular Uptake and Location of RITC-MCNCs

To facilitate CLSM observation, MCNCs were grafted by red RITC (Rhodamine B isothiocyanate) by the similar procedure as described in Chap. 3 for the fabrication of FITC-MCNCs. HeLa cells were seeded into a CLSM-specific cell culture dish with the cell density of 50–60 %, which was cultured in 5 % CO_2 at 37 °C. Then, the cell culture media was replaced with the culture media containing RITC-MCNCs (2 mL, 50 μg/mL). After further co-incubation for 2 h, the cells were washed by PBS for three times. The nuclei of HeLa cells were stained by DAPI. The fluorescent images were acquired by a CLSM equipment. The three-dimensional fluorescence reconstruction of the MCNC-endocytosized HeLa cells were recorded by serial layer scanning of cancer cells along Z-axis and 3D reconstruction of scanned fluorescence images.

4.2.5 In Vivo Evaluation of the HIFU Synergistic Effect of IMNCs, PFH-IMNCs, MCNCs, and PFH-MCNCs Against Rabbit VX2 Xenograft

The in vivo evaluation was conducted on an MRI/HIFU therapy apparatus (Chongqing Key Laboratory of Ultrasound in Medicine and Engineering; Therapeutic frequency: 1.0–1.5 MHz, diameter: 180 mm, focal length: 150 mm; MRI-monitoring apparatus: 1.5 T MRI Magnetom Symphony, Body Matrix/Large Loop Coil). New Zealand white rabbits (2.5–3.0 kg) bearing VX2 liver tumor (2–3 cm) were chosen as the model animal. Typically, PBS (2 mL), MCNCs/PBS (2 mL, [MCNCs] = 30 mg/kg), and PFH-MCNCs/PBS (2 mL, [MCNCs] = 30 mg/kg) were intravenously injected into the rabbit. Before and after the administration for different durations (0, 5, 15, and 30 min), T_1-weighted MRI was acquired. The parameters for T1-weighted MR imaging were TR/RE = 502/12, BW = 185, FOV = 400 $\times$ 400, and SL = 4 mm).

After the T_1-weighted MR imaging for 30 min, HIFU was directly acted on the tumor tissue to evaluate the synergistic effect of nanoparticles. The in vivo HIFU irradiation condition was set as the same as in vitro evaluation (150 W/cm^2, 5 s). After the HIFU treatment, the rabbits were sacrificed and anatomized immediately to determine the coagulated tissue volume. The coagulated tumor tissue volumes were calculated by the following equation: $V = \pi/6 \times L_{max} \times W_{max}^2$ (L_{max}: the maximum length of coagulated tumor tissue, W_{max}: the maximum width of coagulated tumor tissue).

4.3   Results and Discussion

4.3.1   IMNCs as the Synergistic Agents for HIFU Ablation

IMNCs as the HIFU synergistic agents are featured with the following characteristics [13]. First, mesoporous silica nanosystems are one of the most promising inorganic materials. Second, the mesoporous structure provides the diffusion paths for guest molecules. Third, the large hollow cavity of IMNCs can enhance the loading capacity for guest molecules. Last but not least, the introduction of IMNCs into tumor tissues can change the acoustic microenvironment of tissues and enhance the ultrasound-energy deposition subsequently. Therefore, the therapeutic efficiency of focused ultrasound can be substantially improved. Focused ultrasound can produce high temperature, which provides the bases to evaporate the biocompatible PFH molecules with relatively low boiling point (51–59 °C). The PFH molecules are initially encapsulated within the large hollow cavity of IMNCs. After the evaporation, the released and evaporated PFH can form the microbubbles to further enhance the synergistic effect of IMNCs.

IMNCs were synthesized by the developed SDSE strategy, as described in Chap. 2. As shown in Fig. 4.1a, IMNCs possess large hollow interior, which can be distinguished from the contrast differences between the core and shell in TEM image. The well-defined spherical morphology can be directly observed in SEM image (Fig. 4.1b). The HIFU-based therapeutic process was described in Fig. 4.1c. Under the guidance of ultrasound imaging, the emitted focused ultrasound from transducer can be focused into the in vivo targeted tumor tissue to ablate the cancer cells. The typical evaluation approaches of HIFU therapeutic efficiency are based on the ex vivo assessment against degassed bovine liver and in vivo animal tumor xenograft. We firstly used degassed bovine liver as the tissue model to evaluate the synergistic performance of IMNCs for HIFU ablation. During the experiment, different agents were directly injected into the tissue for assessment. When the injection site was found by ultrasound imaging, IMNCs PBS solution (200 μL) was immediately injected into the tissue. Then, HIFU was acted on the injection site (150 W/cm^2, 5 s). After HIFU irradiation, the bovine liver was anatomized to calculate the ablation tissue volume. As shown in Fig. 4.1d, PFH-IMNCs (165.5 mm^3) could cause much larger tissue ablation compared to PBS (32.1 mm^3), PFH/PBS (44.2 mm^3) and IMNCs/PBS (64.9 mm^3), demonstrating the high synergistic efficiency.

Based on the desirable ex vivo results, we further chose rabbits as the model animal to evaluate the in vivo synergistic efficiency of IMNCs for HIFU ablation. PBS, PFH/PBS, IMNCs/PBS, and PFH-IMNCs/PBS (2 mL) were injected into rabbits through ear vein, respectively. The nanoparticles could accumulate into liver because of the uptake of IMNCs by in vivo macrophage cells. Ultrasound imaging was used to monitor the gray changes before and after the HIFU irradiation. As shown in Fig. 4.2, all the experimental groups presented the gray changes after the HIFU irradiation, indicating that there was the coagulation within the

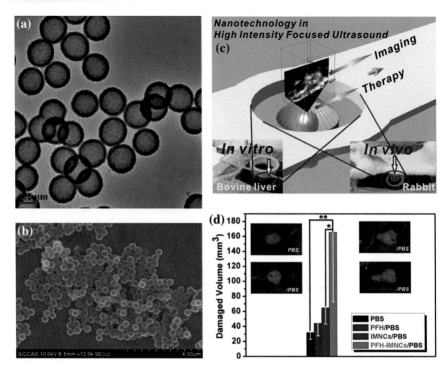

Fig. 4.1 TEM (**a**) and SEM (**b**) images of IMNCs; (**c**) Schematic illustration of the high-intensity focused ultrasound (HIFU) therapeutic principle. The HIFU radiates to the targeted site in the body, and the process is monitored by the outside ultrasound imaging. The ex vivo experiment was conducted using bovine liver as a radiation substrate (the *left* digital picture), while the in vivo experiment was carried out using rabbits as a model animal (the *right* digital picture); **d** Coagulated tissue volume of bovine liver by the intratissue injection of different agents such as PBS (200 μL), PFH/PBS (200 μL), IMNCs/PBS (200 μL) and PFH-IMNCs/PBS (200 μL) under the same irradiation power and duration (150 W/cm^2, 5 s; *$P < 0.1$, **$P < 0.05$). Insets in (**b**) are the macroscopic appearances of bovine liver tissues exposed to HIFU with or without using the synergistic agents. The necrotic tissue is brighter, as can be easily distinguished from their unaffected surroundings. Reproduced with permission from Ref. [13]. © 2012, WILEY-VCH Verlag GmbH & Co. KGaA, Weinheim

tissues by the action of focused ultrasound. Comparatively, the rabbit group receiving PFH-IMNCs/PBS showed much more significant changes of acoustic signals than those of rabbits receiving PBS, PFH/PBS, and IMNCs/PBS. This results gave the direct evidence that the introduction of PFH-IMNCs could easily cause the tumor damage by HIFU irradiation, which was in consistent with the ex vivo results from degassed bovine liver. This result also further indicated that the introduction of PFH-IMNCs could change the acoustic microenvironment of tissue, enhance the ultrasound-energy deposition within tissues, and improve the HIFU therapeutic efficiency.

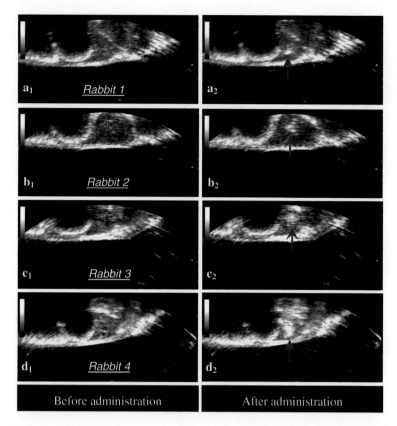

Fig. 4.2 In vivo evaluation of therapeutic efficiency of HIFU by the intravenous injection of different agents into rabbits under the irradiation power of 150 W/cm^2 and duration of 5 s by the ultrasound imaging monitoring outside (a_1 and a_2: PBS (2 mL), b_1 and b_2: PFH/PBS (2 mL), c_1 and c_2: IMNCs/PBS (2 mL), d_1 and d_2: PFH-IMNCs/PBS (2 mL)). Reproduced with permission from Ref. [13]. © 2012, WILEY-VCH Verlag GmbH & Co. KGaA, Weinheim

4.3.2 MCNCs for MRI-Guided HIFU Cancer Surgery

The aforementioned results have demonstrated that FPH-loaded hollow mesoporous nanocapsules (IMNCs) could effectively enhance the HIFU-based ablation efficiency. It is important to note that the positioning of HIFU irradiation also determines the precision and efficiency of HIFU therapy. Before HIFU irradiation, the targeted lesion should be clearly distinguished by various imaging modalities for HIFU action. The precise imaging of tumor tissues could distinguish the boundaries between the normal and abnormal tissue, based on which the boundary could be initially ablated to cut the blood and nutrition supply. This therapeutic modality could maximum ablate the tumors with high efficiency. In addition, the precision of ultrasound positioning could reduce the damage of HIFU

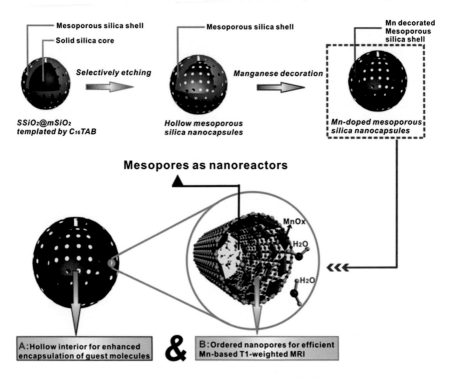

Fig. 4.3 Schematic diagram of the synthetic procedure for MCNCs and their corresponding microstructures. Reproduced with permission from Ref. [14]. © 2011, WILEY-VCH Verlag GmbH & Co. KGaA, Weinheim

to normal tissues, thus, the side effects and pains to patients could be mitigated. All these considerations are based on the high-performance imaging modality.

Herein, we designed a new type of MCNCs at nanoscale for MRI-guided HIFU synergistic therapy [14]. As shown in Fig. 4.3, C_{16}TAB-tempated hollow mesoporous silica nanoparticles were initially synthesized based on the developed SDSE strategy. Then, MnO_4^- ions were introduced to react with C_{16}TAB molecules, by which MnOx nanoparticles could be in-situ generated within mesopores. From the microstructural characteristics, these MCNCs are feature with the following two advantages. On one hand, the large surface area and well-defined mesoporous structure could disperse the Mn paramagnetic center to obtain the high-performance T_1-weighted MRI contrast agents. On the other hand, the large hollow cavity of MCNCs could be used for loading PFH molecules to act as the synergistic agents for HIFU ablation. Therefore, PFH-loaded MCNCs could play the specific roles for MRI-guided HIFU synergistic therapy.

The evolution of MCNCs structure was observed by TEM. We chose highly dispersed hollow mesoporous SiO_2 nanoparticles as the matrix for further MnOx-based multifunctionalization (Fig. 4.4a). Based on soft/hard dual-templating method, $sSiO_2@mSiO_2$ nanoparticles (Fig. 4.4b) were first synthesized. Based on

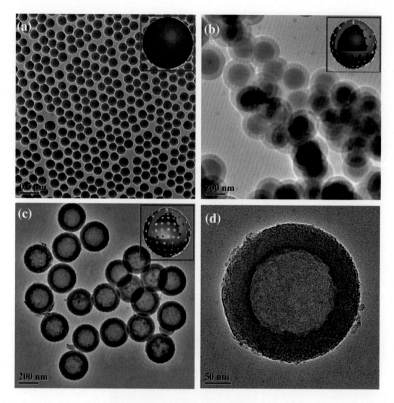

Fig. 4.4 TEM images of solid SiO_2 nanoparticles (**a**), $sSiO_2@mSiO_2$ nanoparticles (**b**) and hollow mesoporous silica nanoparticles (**c** and **d**) at different magnifications

the developed SDSE strategy in Chap. 2, the solid silica core could be selectively etched away to produce highly dispersed HMSNs (Fig. 4.4c, d). The mesopores of HMSNs were templated by $C_{16}TAB$ as the structural-directing agent, and the hollow cavity was templated by solid SiO_2 core as the hard template. The organic micelles formed by $C_{16}TAB$ uniformly distributed within the mesopores. After the introduction of MnO_4^- ions with high oxidizing ability, MnO_4^- ions could in-situ react with $C_{16}TAB$ molecules by redox reaction, by which MnOx nanoparticles could be formed and uniformly dispersed within mesopores. The mesoporous channel acted as the nanoreactor to provide the space for redox reaction. The highly dispersed Mn paramagnetic centers endowed the carrier with high T_1-weighted MRI performance (Fig. 4.5a, b). The high dispersion of Mn element could be clearly distinguished in EDS element mapping images. As shown in Fig. 4.5c–f, Mn elements distributed within the whole matrix without obvious aggregation, indicating that this mesopore-confined growth approach could effectively restrict the formed MnOx nanoparticles within the mesopores, facilitating the exposure of Mn paramagnetic centers to water molecules. The well-defined mesopores made the free diffusion of water molecules possible. Therefore, the

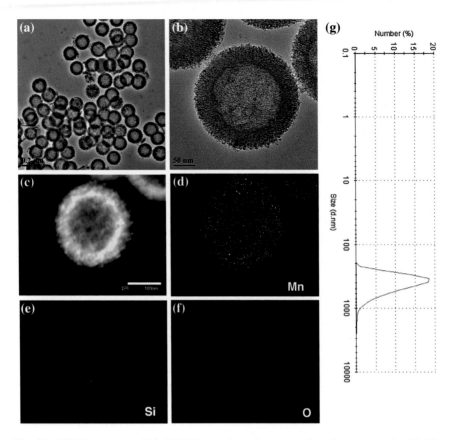

Fig. 4.5 TEM images (**a** and **b**), STEM image (**c**) and corresponding element mapping (**d**: Mn, **e**: Si and **f**: O) of MCNCs; (**g**) The hydrated particle size distribution of MCNCs (after H_2/Ar reduction) in water by dynamic light scattering (DLS) measurement. Reproduced with permission from Ref. [14]. © 2011, WILEY-VCH Verlag GmbH & Co. KGaA, Weinheim

T_1-weighted MRI performance could be enhanced. The Mn amount within MCNCs was determined to be 6.4 % by ICP-AES. DLS results showed that the average particulate size of MCNCs was about 343 nm (Fig. 4.5g). N_2 absorption–desorption technique was used to characterize the mesoporous structure of MCNCs. As shown in Fig. 4.6, MCNCs kept the well-defined mesoporous structure. After the reduction at high temperature, the surface area and pore volume of MCNCs are 468 m^2/g and 0.6 cm^3/g, respectively (Fig. 4.6a). In addition, MCNCs showed the hierarchical mesoporous structure where the average pore sizes are 3.8 and 12.6 nm (Fig. 4.6b). The large mesopores were formed by the chemical etching of the mesopores by mild alkaline solution (Na_2CO_3 solution).

In vitro performance of MCNCs as the contrast agents for T_1-weighted MR imaging was evaluated on a 3.0 T MRI scanning apparatus. The longitudinal relaxation rate (T_1^{-1}) and transverse relaxation rate (T_2^{-1}) as a function of the

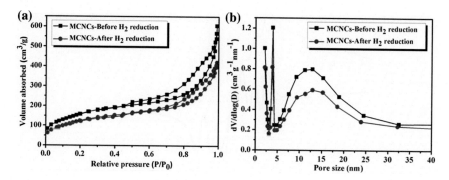

Fig. 4.6 N_2 adsorption–desorption isotherms of MCNCs before and after H_2 reduction (**a**), and the corresponding pore size distributions (**b**)

Mn concentrations in the MCNCs were assessed before and after H_2/Ar reduction. The relaxation rates r_1 of MCNCs before and after H_2/Ar reduction were 0.57 and 1.84 $mM^{-1}\ s^{-1}$ (Fig. 4.7a). The r_2 values increased from initial 19.9 to 42.0 $mM^{-1}\ s^{-1}$ after the H_2/Ar reduction (Fig. 4.7b). The r_1 and r_2 values increased by 3.2 and 2.1 times because of the reduction which was due to the decrease of Mn valence caused by H_2/Ar reduction. Such a valence decrease was also demonstrated by the electron spin resonance (ESR, Fig. 4.8). Such a r_1 value was 4.0, 9.2, 13.2, and 14.3 times higher than those of 7 nm (0.37 $mM^{-1}\ s^{-1}$), 15 nm (0.18 $mM^{-1}\ s^{-1}$), 20 nm (0.13 $mM^{-1}\ s^{-1}$), and 25 nm (0.13 $mM^{-1}\ s^{-1}$) monodispersed manganese oxide nanoparticles, [15, 16], respectively. The main advantage of MCNCs as the T_1-weighted MRI contrast agents was their highly dispersed Mn paramagnetic centers within mesopores, thus increased the chances to intact with water molecules.

Tables 4.1 and 4.2 show the T_1/T_2 values and phantom images of MCNCs in aqueous solution before and after H_2/Ar reduction. It was found that T_1-weighted images of MCNCs aqueous solution became brighter, while T_2-weighted images

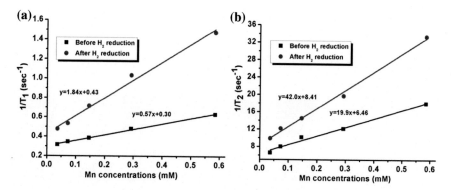

Fig. 4.7 Plots of (**a**) T_1^{-1} and (**b**) T_2^{-1} versus manganese ion concentrations of MCNCs before and after H_2/Ar reduction

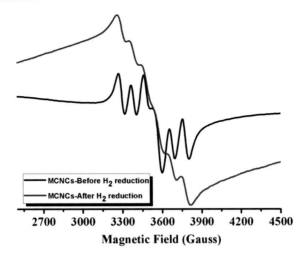

Fig. 4.8 Electron spin resonance (ESR) spectra of MCNCs before and after H_2/Ar reduction. It can be inferred that the increased relaxivities of MCNCs after H_2/Ar reduction are mainly due to the lowed valence of manganese ions under reducing atmosphere (e.g., Mn^{4+}–Mn^{2+} transformation), similar to the valence reduction of Fe ions from Fe_2O_3 to Fe_3O_4 under H_2/Ar atmosphere, which was demonstrated by the higher hyperfine splitting (A) value after H_2/Ar reduction as indicated in ESR spectra of MCNCs

Table 4.1 T_1/T_2 values and phantom images of MCNCs before H_2/Ar reduction

[Mn] (mM)	0	0.037	0.073	0.146	0.293	0.585
T_1 phantom image (*Before*)						
T_1 (ms)	3432	2883	2594	2083	1584	1036
T_2 phantom image (*After*)						
T_2 (ms)	258	125	99	82	55	37

Table 4.2 T_1/T_2 values and phantom images of MCNCs after H_2/Ar reduction

[Mn] (mM)	0	0.037	0.073	0.146	0.293	0.585
T_1 phantom image (*Before*)						
T_1 (ms)	3519	1828	1399	968	677	485
T_2 phantom image (*After*)						
T_2 (ms)	258	82	69	51	30	19

became darker with the increase of Mn concentrations, which indicated that the introduction of MCNCs generated significant T_1 and T_2 contrast-enhanced effects. In addition, MCNCs after H_2/Ar reduction exhibited much lower relaxation time, further demonstrating the enhanced T_1/T_2-weighted MRI performances.

The efficient endocytosis of MCNCs guarantees the promising MRI-guided HIFU synergistic therapy. The endocytosis of MCNCs and intracellular location of MCNCs were further determined by confocal laser scanning microscopy (CLSM). To facilitate CLSM observation, MCNCs were grafted with organic fluorescein RITC with red fluorescence. Two cancer cell lines, HeLa and MCF-7, were chosen to co-incubate with RITC-MCNCs. The remaining nanocapsules were washed by PBS and the fluorescent images of cancer cells were acquired by CLSM. As shown in Fig. 4.9, large amounts of red dots representing FITC-MCNCs could

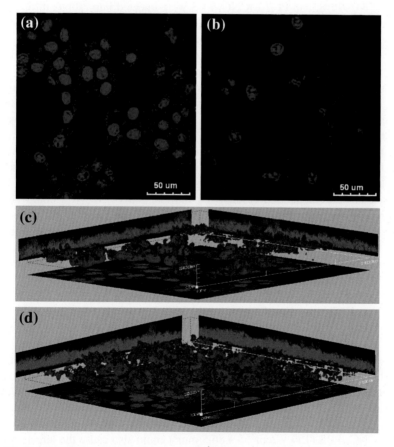

Fig. 4.9 Confocal laser scanning microscopy (CLSM) images of HeLa (**a**) and MCF-7 (**b**) cells after incubation with RITC-MCNCs for 2 h (RITC-MCNCs concentration: 50 μg/mL), and three-dimensional confocal fluorescence reconstructions of MCNCs-endocytosed HeLa (**c**) and MCF-7 (**d**) cells to demonstrate the internalization of nanoparticles within cancer cells. The cell nuclei were stained with DAPI (*blue* fluorescence) and the RITC exhibited the *red* fluorescence

be found within cancer cells. The nuclei of cancer cells were stained with DAPI. Based on the overlap images, it was found that FITC-MCNCs were mainly present within the cytoplasm of cancer cells. No nanocapsules were found in the nuclei, indicating that FITC-MCNCs could enter the nuclei of cancer cells. By three-dimensional fluorescent image reconstruction, it was also demonstrated that the endocytosized FITC-MCNCs were mainly located within the cytoplasm not in the nuclei. Therefore, the CLSM results provided the direct evidence the FITC-MCNCs could be effectively endocytosized into cancer cells.

The high in vitro performance of MCNCs as the contrast agents for T_1-weighted MR imaging encouraged us to explore their in vivo performance. The rabbits bearing VX2 liver tumors were chosen as the animal tumor xenograft for in vivo experiment. To facilitate the subsequent assessment of MRI-guided HIFU synergistic therapy, the apparatus for in vivo experiment was a 1.5 T MRI system. PBS, MCNCs/PBS, and PFH-MCNCs/PBS were injected into rabbits through ear vein, respectively. After the administration of PBS, the liver tissue and tumor had no obvious signal variation (Fig. 4.10a_1–a_4). Comparatively, the significant MRI signal changes could be clearly distinguished in the liver and tumor of rabbits receiving MCNCs/PBS (Fig. 4.10b_1–b_4) and PFH-MCNCs/PBS (Fig. 4.10c_1–c_4). Such a T_1-weighed MRI signal enhancement was due to the contrast-enhanced effect of MCNCs, which could accumulate into liver by the uptake of macrophages. The MRI signal enhancement further indicated that the nanocapsules could enter the tumor tissues. Especially, the boundary between the normal liver tissue and tumor became much clearer after the introduction of MCNCs, which could facilitate the subsequent HIFU positioning, enhance the targeting effect of HIFU therapy, and mitigate the side effects.

Based on aforementioned results, the introduction of MCNCs could act as the contrast agents for T1-weighted MR imaging of tumor tissue. The following research focused on the synergistic effect of MCNCs for HIFU ablation. Similar to the evaluating procedure for IMNCs, the degassed bovine liver was used as the model tissue for ex vivo assessment. The real-time ultrasound imaging was applied for monitoring the whole procedure. When the injection site was found by ultrasound imaging, different agents were immediately injected into the bovine liver. Then, HIFU was directly acted on the injection site. Finally, the bovine liver was anatomized for calculating the coagulation volume of liver tissue. As shown in Fig. 4.11a, the coagulation volume of tissues after receiving MCNCs/PBS was larger than the control PBS group. Importantly, the injection of PFH-MCNCs/PBS (150 W/cm^2, 5 s 86.5 mm^3; 250 W/cm^2, 5 s 153.1 mm^3) could induce much larger coagulation volume of tissues than the tissues receiving PBS (150 W/cm^2, 5 s 31.7 mm^3; 250 W/cm^2, 5 s 66.6 mm^3) and MCNCs/PBS (150 W/cm^2, 5 s 43.7 mm^3, 250 W/cm^2, 5 s 109.3 mm^3). It is noted that the administration of PFH-MCNCs/PBS (150 W/cm^2, 5 s 86.5 mm^3) could also cause the larger coagulation tissue volume at low irradiation power than the control PBS at high irradiation power (250 W/cm^2, 5 s 66.6 mm^3). This high therapeutic effect indicated that HIFU could exert the similar or even higher therapeutic outcome at low power with the assistance by the introduction of PFH-MCNCs/PBS as the synergistic

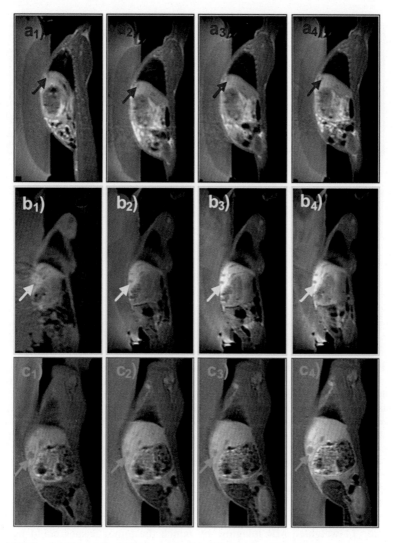

Fig. 4.10 In vivo T_1-weighted MR imaging of rabbits bearing VX2 liver tumor before (**a₁**, **b₁**, and **c₁**) and after (5 min: **a₂**, **b₂**, and **c₂**; 15 min: **a₃**, **b₃**, and **c₃**; 30 min: **a₄**, **b₄**, and **c₄**) administration of different agents (PBS: **a₁–a₄**; MCNCs/PBS: **b₁–b₄**; PFH-MCNCs/PBS: **c₁–c₄**) via ear vein. *Arrows* indicate the tumor. Reproduced with permission from Ref. [14]. © 2011, WILEY-VCH Verlag GmbH & Co. KGaA, Weinheim

agent, which could avoid the damage to normal tissues of HIFU at high therapeutic power.

As shown in Fig. 4.11b, the combination of ultrasound transducer and MRI magnetic field can construct an integrated therapeutic system for MRI-guided HIFU cancer surgery. The introduction of MCNCs could first act as the contrast

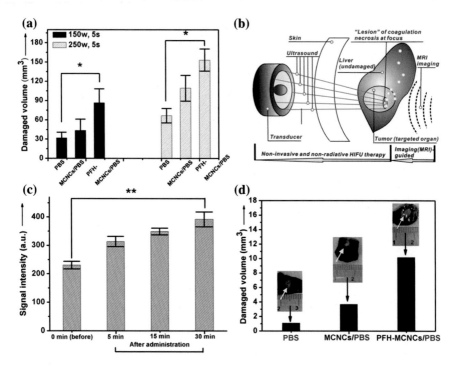

Fig. 4.11 **a** Coagulated tissue volumes of degassed bovine liver by the intratissue injection of different agents of PBS (200 μL), MCNCs/PBS (200 μL) and PFH-MCNCs/PBS (200 μL) under the same irradiation power and duration (150 W/cm^2, 5 s and 250 W/cm^2, 5 s; *$P < 0.05$); **b** Technical principle of MRI-guided HIFU for the surgery of hepatic neoplasm in rabbits; **c** T$_1$-weighted MRI signal intensities of tumor tissue before and after intravenous administration of PFH-MCNCs/PBS (**$P < 0.005$); **d** In vivo coagulated necrotic tumor volume by MRI-guided HIFU exposure under the irradiation power of 150 w/cm^2 and duration of 5 s in rabbit liver tumors after receiving different agents via ear vein (*inset* digital pictures of tumor tissue after HIFU exposure). Reproduced with permission from Ref. [14]. © 2011, WILEY-VCH Verlag GmbH & Co. KGaA, Weinheim

agents for T1-weighted MR imaging, by which the tumor tissues could be precisely positioned. The ultrasound generated by the transducer could be focused onto the tumor part with the assistance by MR imaging. The accumulation of MCNCs within tumor changed the acoustic microenvironment of tumor, enhances the ultrasound-energy deposition within the tissue, and improves the HIFU therapeutic efficiency. Herein, MCNCs acted not only as the MRI contrast agents, but also as the synergistic agent to enhance the HIFU therapeutic outcome. To further assess the in vivo performance of MCNCs for HIFU synergistic therapy, the rabbits bearing VX2 liver tumor were chosen as the animal model. MCNCs easily accumulated into tumor tissues by passive EPR effect. After intravenous administration of PBS, MCNCs/PBS and PFH-MCNCs/PBS for 30 min, the tumors and

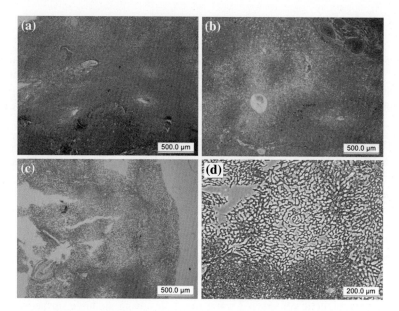

Fig. 4.12 Pathological examinations of related tumor tissues after HIFU ablation via intravenous administration of PBS (**a**), MCNCs/PBS (**b**) and PFH-MCNCs/PBS (**c** and **d**) based on MRI guidance

the boundary could be clearly distinguished in MR images (Fig. 4.11c), by which HIFU could be precisely acted onto the tumor. After HIFU irradiation (150 W/cm^2, 5 s), the rabbits were anatomized for calculating the coagulated tumor volume. It was found that there existed the significant differences among different experimental groups (Fig. 4.11d). Especially, the coagulation tumor volume of rabbits receiving PFH-MCNCs/PBS reached 10.2 mm^3, much larger than PBS (1.1 mm^3), and MCNCs/PBS (3.7 mm^3). This result strongly demonstrated that the employment of PFH-MCNCs could be used for MRI-guided HIFU synergistic therapy, which was in consistent with ex vivo evaluations against bovine liver.

Figure 4.12 shows the hematoxylin–eosin (HE) staining results of tumor tissues after HIFU ablation. It was found that the tumor receiving PBS (Fig. 4.12a) or MCNCs/PBS (Fig. 4.12b) showed the compact and aggregated cell distributions accompanying a few denatured cancer cells. Comparatively, the tumor tissues receiving PFH-MCNCs/PBS exhibited destructed cancer cells, large vacuoles, and irregular widening of tumor tissues (Fig. 4.12c, d), indicating the high therapeutic efficiency of HIFU assisted by the introduction of PFH-MCNCs/PBS [17, 18]. The high therapeutic efficiency could be attributed to the changed acoustic microenvironment of tumor tissues. In addition, the encapsulated PFH could be evaporated by HIFU thermal effect, which could induce the cavitation effect to improve the HIFU ablation outcome.

4.4 Conclusions

In this chapter, inorganic mesoporous silica nanocapsules (IMNCs) were introduced into HIFU synergistic therapy which was systematically evaluated both ex vivo and in vivo. In addition, MCNCs with multifunctionalization were designed and fabricated for MRI-guided HIFU synergistic therapy. Several results are summarized as follows.

(1) The ex vivo and in vivo results have confirmed that the introduction of IMNCs could effectively change the acoustic microenvironment of tissues, enhance the ultrasound-energy deposition into targeted tissue, and improve the HIFU surgical outcome. In addition, the introduction of PFH with low boiling point into the hollow cavity of IMNCs further enhanced the HIFU ablation efficiency.
(2) By in-situ dispersion of MnOx nanoparticles into the mesopores, a high-performance T_1-weighted MRI contrast agents could be fabricated with much higher imaging capability than that of traditional MnO nanoparticles. The high MRI performance was due to the maximized interactions between Mn paramagnetic centers and water molecules using the large surface area of MCNCs. MCNCs-based MRI contrast agents showed excellent imaging outcome in T_1-weighted in vivo MR imaging of rabbit VX2 liver tumor.
(3) By intravenous administration of MCNCs into rabbits bearing VX2 liver tumor xenograft, MRI could be used for precise positioning of the tumors. By further loading PFH into MCNCs, the organic-inorganic nanocapsules could act as the synergistic agents for enhancing the HIFU therapeutic efficiency. Both ex vivo and in vivo results have confirmed this issue.

Noninvasive medicine is the main promising therapeutic modality for cancer treatment. Mesoporous materials can not only be used in HIFU cancer surgery, but also they are promising candidates to enhance the therapeutic efficiency of other therapeutic modalities, such as microwave therapy and radiotherapy. The large hollow cavity and well-defined mesopores of multifunctional mesoporous nanocapsules can further encapsulate the anticancer drug molecules to realize the combination of chemotherapy and HIFU therapy. This new therapeutic strategy will provide more therapeutic protocols and ideas to realize the tumor therapy with high efficiency and safety.

References

1. Bailey MR, Khokhlova VA, Sapozhnikov OA, Kargl SG, Crum LA (2003) Physical mechanisms of the therapeutic effect of ultrasound—(a review). Acoust Phys 49(4):369–388
2. Kennedy JE, ter Haar GR, Cranston D (2003) High intensity focused ultrasound: surgery of the future? Br J Radiol 76(909):590–599
3. Hynynen K (2010) MRI-guided focused ultrasound treatments. Ultrasonics 50(2):221–229

4. Schmitz AC, Gianfelice D, Daniel BL, Mali W, van den Bosch M (2008) Image-guided focused ultrasound ablation of breast cancer: current status, challenges, and future directions. Eur Radiol 18(7):1431–1441

5. Huber PE, Jenne JW, Rastert R, Simiantonakis I, Sinn HP, Strittmatter HJ, von Fournier D, Wannenmacher MF, Debus J (2001) A new noninvasive approach in breast cancer therapy using magnetic resonance imaging-guided focused ultrasound surgery. Cancer Res 61(23):8441–8447

6. Park JI, Jagadeesan D, Williams R, Oakden W, Chung SY, Stanisz GJ, Kumacheva E (2010) Microbubbles loaded with nanoparticles: a route to multiple imaging modalities. ACS Nano 4(11):6579–6586

7. Deelman LE, Decleves AE, Rychak JJ, Sharma K (2010) Targeted renal therapies through microbubbles and ultrasound. Adv Drug Deliv Rev 62(14):1369–1377

8. Nakatsuka MA, Hsu MJ, Esener SC, Cha JN, Goodwin AP (2011) DNA-coated microbubbles with biochemically tunable ultrasound contrast activity. Adv Mater 23(42):4908–4912

9. Schutt EG, Klein DH, Mattrey RM, Riess JG (2003) Injectable microbubbles as contrast agents for diagnostic ultrasound imaging: the key role of perfluorochemicals. Angew Chem-Int Edit 42(28):3218–3235

10. Lindner JR (2004) Microbubbles in medical imaging: current applications and future directions. Nat Rev Drug Discov 3(6):527–532

11. Oerlemans C, Deckers R, Storm G, Hennink WE, Nijsen JFW (2013) Evidence for a new mechanism behind HIFU-triggered release from liposomes. J Control Release 168(3):327–333

12. Fang XL, Chen C, Liu ZH, Liu PX, Zheng NF (2011) A cationic surfactant assisted selective etching strategy to hollow mesoporous silica spheres. Nanoscale 3(4):1632–1639

13. Chen Y, Gao Y, Chen HR, Zeng DP, Li YP, Zheng YY, Li FQ, Ji XF, Wang X, Chen F, He QJ, Zhang LL, Shi JL (2012) Engineering inorganic nanoemulsions/nanoliposomes by fluoride-silica chemistry for efficient delivery/co-delivery of hydrophobic agents. Adv Funct Mater 22(8):1586–1597

14. Chen Y, Chen HR, Sun Y, Zheng YY, Zeng DP, Li FQ, Zhang SJ, Wang X, Zhang K, Ma M, He QJ, Zhang LL, Shi JL (2011) Multifunctional mesoporous composite nanocapsules for highly efficient mri-guided high-intensity focused ultrasound cancer surgery. Angew Chem-Int Edit 50(52):12505–12509

15. Na HB, Lee JH, An KJ, Park YI, Park M, Lee IS, Nam DH, Kim ST, Kim SH, Kim SW, Lim KH, Kim KS, Kim SO, Hyeon T (2007) Development of a T-1 contrast agent for magnetic resonance imaging using MnO nanoparticles. Angew Chem-Int Edit 46(28):5397–5401

16. Pan DPJ, Schmieder AH, Wickline SA, Lanza GM (2011) Manganese-based MRI contrast agents: past, present, and future. Tetrahedron 67(44):8431–8444

17. Kaneko Y, Maruyama T, Takegami K, Watanabe T, Mitsui H, Hanajiri K, Nagawa HA, Matsumoto Y (2005) Use of a microbubble agent to increase the effects of high intensity focused ultrasound on liver tissue. Eur Radiol 15(7):1415–1420

18. Takegami K, Kaneko Y, Watanabe T, Watanabe S, Maruyama T, Matsumoto Y, Nagawa H (2005) Heating and coagulation volume obtained with high-intensity focused ultrasound therapy: Comparison of perflutren protein-type A microspheres and MRX-133 in rabbits. Radiology 237(1):132–136

Chapter 5
Summary and Outlook

5.1 Summary

This thesis aims to develop multifunctional mesoporous silica-based drug delivery nanosystems for biomedical applications based on nano-synthetic chemistry. Multifunctionalization of mesoporous silica nanoparticles includes surface grafting, mesopore modification, hollow-structure construction and the integration of several functionalization strategies. The structure-property relationships of the as-synthesized multifunctional mesoporous silica nanoparticles have been revealed. Furthermore, their extensive applications for enhanced drug loading, improved therapeutic efficiency, molecular imaging and HIFU cancer surgery have been systematically investigated. The main conclusions of this thesis are summarized as follows.

Construction of hollow mesoporous silica nanoparticles (HMSNs) for anti-cancer drug delivery

We proposed a new "structural difference-based selective etching" (SDSE) strategy to design and synthesize HMSNs. Different from traditional methods based on the compositional difference between the core and shell to fabricate the hollow cavity, this method utilizes the structural difference between the core and shell while the compositions are the same, by which the inner core can be selectively etched away at nanoscale. FTIR and ^{29}Si MAS NMR characterizations demonstrate such a structural difference originates from the variations of condensation degree of the silica precursor. Based on the structural difference, HMSNs with controllable particle sizes (60, 180 and 360 nm) have been successfully synthesized by either Na_2CO_3 or ammonia etching. In addition, rattle-type hollow $SiO_2@mSiO_2$ nanoparticles could be fabricated by controlling the etching procedure. This strategy could be further extended to synthesize multifunctional $M@mSiO_2$ (M = Au, Fe_2O_3, Fe_3O_4) nanorattles with inorganic nanocrystals as the core, mesoporous silica as the shell and large hollow cavity in between. The achieved HMSNs with large hollow cavity showed enhanced drug-loading

© Springer-Verlag Berlin Heidelberg 2016
Y. Chen, *Design, Synthesis, Multifunctionalization and Biomedical Applications of Multifunctional Mesoporous Silica-Based Drug Delivery Nanosystems*, Springer Theses, DOI 10.1007/978-3-662-48622-1_5

capacity. Their loading amount for doxorubicin (DOX) was as high as 1222 mg/g. Importantly, DOX-loaded HMSNs exhibited much higher anticancer efficiency compared to free DOX. In addition, HMSNs possess excellent blood compatibility and low cytotoxicity.

Construction of multifunctional HMSNs for concurrent diagnostic imaging and anticancer drug delivery

Based on SESE strategy for the fabrication of hollow mesoporous silica-based nanoparticles, a series of multifunctional $M@mSiO_2$(M = Fe_2O_3, Fe_3O_4, Au) nanocapsules have been successfully constructed. The magnetic Fe_3O_4 core of $Fe_3O_4@mSiO_2$ nanocapsules could be used as the contrast agents for T_2-weighted MRI (r_2 = 137.8 mM^{-1} s^{-1}). In addition, the large hollow cavity of $Fe_3O_4@mSiO_2$ nanocapsules endows the carrier with high drug-loading capacity (DOX: 20 % loading amount and ~100 % loading efficiency). MTT results showed that the encapsulated DOX within $Fe_3O_4@mSiO_2$ nanocapsules possessed much higher cytotoxicity compared to free DOX. The biocompatibility evaluation demonstrated that the prepared $Fe_3O_4@mSiO_2$ nanocapsules had excellent blood compatibility (low hemolytic and coagulation effects) and low cytotoxicity. For biomedical applications of $Au@mSiO_2$ nanorattles, Gd–Si-DTPA was successfully grafted into the mesopores of $Au@mSiO_2$ nanorattles, which could act as the dual-mode contrast agents for dark-field light-scattering cell labeling and T_1-weighted MR imaging. The relaxation rate r_1 was as high as 7.43 mM^{-1} s^{-1}.

Hollow mesoporous silica-based nanosystems for MRI-guided HIFU synergistic therapy

Multifunctional HMSNs were for the first time introduced into non-invasive HIFU cancer surgery. It was demonstrated that PFH-loaded HMSNs could effectively enhance the efficiency of HIFU ablation. Further MnOx multifunctionalization could act as the concurrent contrast agents and synergistic agents for MRI-guided HIFU ablation, which effectively solve the critical issues of efficiency and biosafety during HIFU ablation. After intravenous administration of MCNCs into rabbits bearing VX2 liver tumor, the tumor tissue and the boundary between tumor and normal tissue could be clearly distinguished. The relaxation time r_1 was 1.84 mM^{-1} s^{-1}. After further loading of PFH into the large hollow cavity, the composite nanocapsules could enhance the ultrasound-energy deposition within the tumor tissue to enhance the HIFU ablation outcome, which was demonstrated both ex vivo and in vivo. The coagulation tumor volume of rabbits receiving PFH-MCNCs/PBS was 10.2 mm^3, much larger than PBS (1.1 mm^3) and MCNCs/PBS (3.7 mm^3).

5.2 Outlook

This thesis controlled the microstructure, composition and morphology of HMSNs to achieve mesoporous silica-based biomaterials with higher performance in biomedicine, which substantially broadens the application fields of traditional mesoporous silica nanoparticles. Systematic researches have confirmed that multifunctionalization of HMSNs can not only enhance the drug-loading capacity, but also endows the carrier with diagnostic-imaging capability (e.g., MRI, fluorescent imaging and ultrasound imaging). These elaborately designed and fabricated nanocarriers could effectively solve the critical issues of biomedicine. The researches in this thesis provide more methodologies and ideas for the applications of mesoporous materials in biomedicine. However, the current researches are mainly concentrated on the design and fabrication of multifunctional mesoporous nanosystems to meet the requirements of specific biomedical applications. The preliminary biosafety evaluations have been conducted. Systematic biological evaluations are still rare, and much more work should be conducted in the near future to promote the clinical applications of mesoporous silica biomaterials.

(1) Based on SDSE strategy to fabricate HMSNs, the surface of HMSNs should be further modified with targeting moieties to enhance the accumulation of HMSNs within tumor tissues, which is the crucial issue to improve the chemotherapeutic efficiency of HMSNs.

(2) The microstructures and compositions of multifunctional HMSNs should be further optimized to enhance the HIFU therapeutic efficiency, such as the positioning and efficiency. The targeting transportation of multifunctional HMSNs should also be realized.

(3) Systematic researches should be conducted to evaluate the biosafety of HMSNs and multifunctional HMSNs, such as the biodistribution, excretion, histo/hemocompatibility. The high biocompatibility of HMSNs or multifunctional HMSNs guarantees their further clinical translations.

Fig. 5.1 Road map for the design and fabrication of mesoporous silica-based multifunctional drug delivery systems

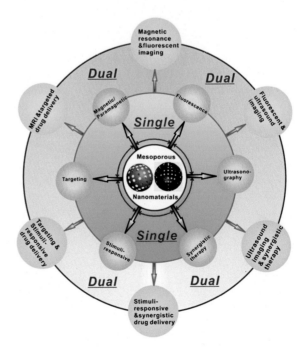

Finally, we propose a simple but versatile principle to design and fabricate multifunctional mesoporous silica-based drug delivery nanosystems. As shown in Fig. 5.1, various multifunctional modules can be integrated into mesoporous silica nanosystems, such as magnetic, fluorescent, targeting, synergistic-therapeutic, stimuli-responsive functions. Single multifunctionalization can be achieved by such a integration. Furthermore, two modules can be integrated into mesoporous silica to fabricate dual-functionalized mesoporous silica. Multifunctional mesoporous silica with even more functions can be achieved. It does not mean that integrating more functions is better. More functions required stricter biosafety evaluations, which means that the biosafety is low. Such a multifunctionalization strategy should base on the practical clinical requirements.

The biomedical applications of mesoporous silica nanosystems are still at the preliminary stage. Much more systematic researches should be further conducted to promote their clinical applications. In addition to fabricate various mesoporous silica-based theranostics, more attentions should be focused on the biological effects of mesoporous nanosystems. The biosafety should be assessed in detail, including histo/hemocompatibility, degradability, excretion, biodistribution, etc. Different animal models should be used to evaluate the biosafety of these nanocarriers, which can guarantee the further clinical translations. With the development of science and technology, we strongly believe that more multifunctional intelligent nanoparticles will be designed in the near future, and these nanoparticles will respond to the external demand to benefit the human health.

Printed in the United States
By Bookmasters